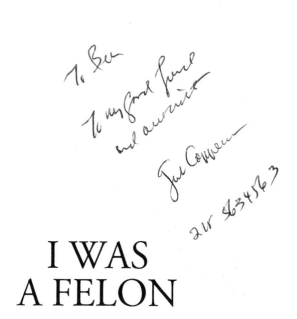

I WAS
A FELON

**STOP DANGEROUS CLIMATE
ENGINEERING**

GEOENGINEERINGWATCH
.ORG

D1564016

I WAS
A FELON

*And Other Stories From the
Life of a Woman Doctor*

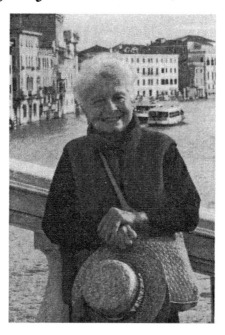

Gertrude Copperman, M.D.

To order additional copies of this book, contact:
Xlibris Corporation
1-888-795-4274
www.Xlibris.com
Orders@Xlibris.com
27233

CONTENTS

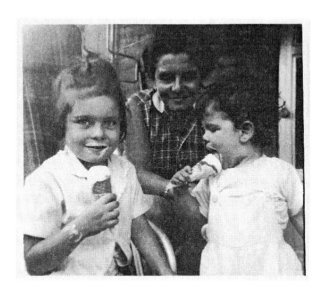

To my wonderful, encouraging, and loving daughters,
Barbara and Joan

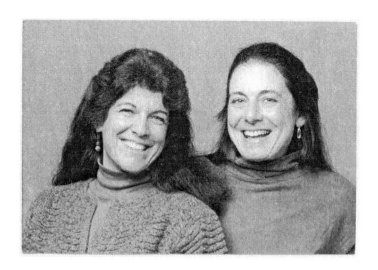

Better pass boldly into that other world in the full glory of some passion than fade and wither dismally with age.

—James Joyce

Introduction

Practice Before

My lifetime in medicine began in 1952. These last fifty-plus years have witnessed amazing advances in patient care. Antibiotics, steroids, chemotherapy, radiation therapy, MRIs, CAT scans, bone scans . . . all contribute to better health and longevity.

Many benefits, however, are disappearing because of the restrictive changes in the field today. The growth of managed care agencies (HMOs) has become synonymous with bureaucracy that results in the loss of physicians' autonomy, shrinking reimbursements, heavier patient loads, less time permitted for each appointment, decreased coverage for patient testing, and poorer overall medical care. Soaring malpractice premiums are compelling physicians to retire early or move to states with lower premiums. Doctors are forced to order unnecessary tests for their own protection in the practice of "defensive" medicine.

In addition to technical advances in medical care and changes in health insurance, the profile of physicians has also changed dramatically in the past half-century. When I entered medical school in 1945, only 6 percent of a freshman class was female. Today women make up 49 percent of medical school students across the country. In some schools, such as the University of Pennsylvania, the percentage is as high as 57 percent. The small increase in female enrollment in the 1970s was due in part to the woman's movement, but the large numbers of women entering medicine today also reflect the declining attraction of the field for men. In 1955, eleven students applied for one seat in a medical school, but today only two apply for each seat. A doctor's declining income has a certain effect as well, especially because the average debt incurred for medical training is $103,800.

The level of patient care, the time spent with patient and family, and involvement in their emotional as well as medical life, are fast disappearing. In fact, they are hardly recognizable compared to my medical practice. So many of my experiences can no longer be duplicated in today's medical world. My intention in writing these stories has been to capture those experiences before they are forgotten. I was fortunate to be part of a generation when doctors could afford to take time to get to know their patients, their family, and their community. The depth of our relationships and some unique incidents—some funny, some sad, some amazing—recall the kind of doctor-patient relationship now lost. Most of the stories in this collection are directly related to my medical education and practice, but a few stories describe other unusual experiences in my life.

—Gertrude Copperman, M.D.
May, 2004

1

Progress Reversed

"NYU Honors Those It Once Punished 60 Years Later"
That headline in the Philadelphia *Inquirer* on May 6, 2001, reminds me of a significant high school event. The article reports that seven students had been suspended six decades earlier for protesting a policy that benched NYU's African American athletes whenever an opposing college objected to playing with them. This occurred six years before Jackie Robinson integrated major league baseball, fourteen years before Rosa Parks sat down in the white section of a Montgomery, Alabama, bus, and twenty years before Dr. Martin Luther King Jr.'s "I Have A Dream" speech.

In 1940 many northern schools had such "gentlemen's agreements" with their mostly white counterparts. NYU's suspended seven, named the Bates Seven after the benched star fullback, transferred to other colleges, finished their educations, and became professors, teachers, social workers, and physicians. These early leaders were described as having significant student support at the time, but it took the university sixty years to recognize their message and virtue.

In 1939, a year before the NYU event, I was a student at the Philadelphia High School for Girls, the best girls' public academic high school in the city. A fair number of African American students were enrolled. We were comfortably integrated, with admissions from every neighborhood in Philadelphia. All groups were well represented academically and in the after-school clubs. Sports were an important scheduled activity for most of us. We had integrated after-school dances with the local all-boys Central High School.

There were no problems or friction because of color, race, or religion until the planning of the graduating class prom.

Mabel, our senior class president, had gorgeous skin unlike us untreated pimply adolescents. She was blond, a WASP, and came from a prominent family with the proper social connections to reserve the upper-class Bellevue Stratford Hotel at a very low price for our prom. One problem: African Americans were not admitted as guests to this fancy all-white establishment.

At this time in Philadelphia, African American women were mainly employed as domestics or nannies and never as saleswomen even in the cheap stores like Woolworth's Five & Ten. African American men worked as janitors, porters, kitchen help, and in all sorts of unskilled jobs. There were few Horatio Algers, George Washington Carvers, W. E.B. Duboises, and Paul Robesons, though the last was born in Philadelphia. Those who made it into the so-called higher ranks were considered the exceptions.

Discrimination was widely accepted in the 1930s, but not by all of us. And not in my high school. A group of seniors objected vociferously to the proposed prom site. Enmities sparked as we girls took sides. Some of our African American friends were initially reluctant to join us. They didn't want to appear belligerent, or were afraid to team up with us liberals not of the mainstream. Perhaps some didn't trust us:

"Why are you taking up our fight? What's in it for you? You liberals are just using us."

Eventually their objections were almost universally overcome by our longstanding friendships, our previous three years of close involvement, and our sincerity. Then ensued endless discussions, plans for strategy, investigating other sites—we formed a solid working constituency. We met almost weekly after school to move the prom to a place where all might attend.

We won. The prom was held at an integrated country club, one of just a few at the time. Hollow victory it was, though. The ill feelings and rancorous arguments of the year destroyed the thrill and pleasure of the event for me. Instead of attending the prom, I chose to take my first trip to New York that weekend—to the exciting World's Fair and my first ride on the top of an open double-decker bus.

What a shock to cross the George Washington Bridge, a huge span in the air, the biggest bridge I had ever seen, arcing up in the sky. On the shore below, hundreds of grayish dirty men, poorly dressed, dejected, were just sitting around smoking. They were housed in shacks made of cardboard and old packing crates, with roofs of discarded tin scraps. My first exposure to "Hoovervilles." This scene of poverty, squalor, and deprivation reminded me of earlier Depression years under President Herbert Hoover when I had seen well-dressed young and middle-aged men selling huge red apples from street corner carts. I was too young then to appreciate their plight but was struck by their unlikely attire as they tended their street carts. My mother told me that the government supplied the apples to unemployed men to provide them some income.

The river men I saw on prom weekend also reminded me of the bread line marchers, unemployed desperate, hungry men who went to Washington where they were fired upon with live ammunition by government forces trying to disperse them. As I thought of the tragic disfranchising of these people and the horrible way of handling them, the past year of weekly high school confrontations and my personal reward of a trip to New York seemed so petty.

Many decades later we do not have Hoovervilles, but we have large numbers of unemployed: 74 million, from factory workers to investment brokers [N.Y. T. March 2003]. We still have undereducated citizens and homeless street people. And the struggle still continues for the rights of non-whites. The reminder of the NYU Seven marks the real progress our society has made since 1939, but we still have far to go, as another newspaper headline testifies:

Friday, May 2, 2003, *"Georgians Plan Whites-Only Prom Party"*

2

In the Beginning

Rank odors and acrid fumes seep under the heavy wooden doors at the end of a dimly lit, airless hallway leading to a closed chamber. My gut is starting to roil. Is it the stench or the anticipation?

I am one of sixty anxious women entering medical school. For the first time, we are wearing our immaculate, stiff, long white coats. We almost look like doctors. We troop into a bright room where strong, unshielded bulbs concentrate light on fifteen naked formaldehyde-soaked stiffs. They are arranged on parallel rows of tables with their feet facing the wall.

We are unprepared for this horrific scene and our reaction is uncontrollable. We dash as a single body to open all the windows. Gasping loudly, we inhale the fresh outside air. We then turn, slowly and reluctantly, in groups of four to our assigned cadaver who will become our daily companion for the next six months.

Fortunately the face has been molded into a rigid emotionless mask, not at all gruesome, not mimicking the "scream" that I had expected. Without sensitivity or modesty, each unwrapped body lies expectantly, splayed out, legs apart, drenched in formaldehyde.

Lucy approaches her table, gets within two feet, turns, and bolts from the room. We hear her retching as she races down the hall toward the restroom. Eventually she rejoins her group, but over the next several weeks Lucy intermittently turns green and runs to the restroom. She always returns, shaken and pale, and gamely resumes her place with her foursome. After a few weeks, her condition forces her to leave. It is not the cadaverous stench but a difficult first trimester of pregnancy that explains her sensitivity. Lucy is the only student we lose in our first year.

The rising formaldehyde vapors burn. Our eyes tear and our hands chap for the next six months. Every day begins in the human gross anatomy lab. "Gross" indeed. Afternoons are spent in chemistry, pathology, and physiology. Each professor, asserting his or her subject to be the most important, fuels our mounting anxiety and night work. Professors' competition, their vying for importance by piling on work, is about to destroy us. We are so overwhelmed that we finally appeal to the dean to have exams spaced more rationally. Our wonderful, empathic Dr. Marion Fay responds by making our lives and exam schedules more reasonable in their timing but not in their difficulty.

My class becomes a strongly supportive, interactive group, helpful and caring of each other. Perhaps it's because we are all women, or perhaps we are starting early to be the caring persons that our chosen profession requires.

Our study groups last until 1 A.M. We rise at 6 A.M. to start the next day. Physiology, the course I most enjoy, is the real introduction to the study of medicine. But we suffer discomfort from visits a few times a year of anti-vivisection societies that actively protest our experimentation on animals. Yet we treat our animals humanely. They are well anaesthetized and feel no discomfort. These animal experiments provide the means by which we can learn the behavior and mechanisms of the human body. At the end of the experiments, they are sacrificed painlessly and feel nothing.

My physiology lab partner and friend, Mimi, and I are appalled to overhear a member of the protest group say, "They should better use Jews and blacks for these experiments." This remark is even more frightening because this is the 1940s, the decade of war against Nazi Germany. It prompts Mimi to tell me of an incident that occurred at the University of Wisconsin where she was one of the few Jewish students three years earlier. A student approached Mimi, who has a dark complexion and curly hair, and separated her hair over her forehead to see if she had horns. What ignorance!

We name our stiff Sally and use her to develop our special areas of expertise. My best friend Ruthie becomes our nerve dissection expert. Her dissections are so exquisite that she should become a surgeon. As the athlete of the group, I become the expert on the origin and insertion of muscles.

After a few weeks, we fortunately become desensitized to the smell, the drying effect of the formaldehyde on our hands, and the coarse, crawly feeling of our assigned bodies. Still we carry the anatomy lab's odor on our hair, skin, and clothes for the next six months despite showers and laundry.

The intricacies of dissection, nomenclature, and volume of knowledge to absorb are overwhelming, but somehow we return to Sally each day with decreased anxiety. We are slowly learning to live in this constant state of unending tasks, too much to learn, too much to accomplish in too short a time—and with too little sleep. Our diet is as haphazard as the rest of our life. We snack throughout the day but not in the anatomy lab. In the early days of the term, we cannot even manage to leave the lab after morning dissection to go to the lunchroom.

Fifty years later we remember many insignificant but humorous experiences of that stressful first year. For example: Jan has a particular problem in her testicular dissection until she devises a priaptic solution. She encircles the glans with a string and loops it over the light fixture hanging from the ceiling, thus maintaining the penis in a constant state of engorged erection. This unrelieved "hard on" provides an amusing sight to greet us each morning. Jan's solution works well until our male instructor takes umbrage. He feels it either personally painful or inappropriate, and the erection comes down. Pearl then has to hold the penis for Jan while she dissects the scrotum.

We form nightly study groups that meet at each other's apartments. Ruthie lives on a narrow lane within convenient walking distance to school. Her street is lined with tall old trees, heavily limbed with densely leafed branches that hide the street lamps. Betsy is accosted early one evening as she walks alone to Ruthie's apartment. She runs up the stairs, panting, and throws herself on Ruthie's couch.

"Thank heaven for *Gray's Anatomy*. I'll never complain about its weight again," Betsy blurts out. "I clobbered the guy on the head with it when he tried to grab me. He staggered and I ran off!" *Gray's Anatomy*, our very heavy Bible, our daily reference tome, has taken on a new role as Betsy's protector.

This first year is both the most difficult and the best of my many years in school. Despite the long hours of study, the persistent anxiety, the constant fatigue, and lack of sleep, we do have some fun—especially my husband, who offers his body to my classmates so they can practice physical diagnosis. Our hospital is still called a "women's hospital," where most patients are women and children. We have few male patients in the clinic. My husband, happy to act the patient's role, enjoys so many enthusiastic women doing a hands-on examination. Some male students from other medical schools occasionally join our study groups, but Rube is not handled by them—his choice and theirs. He only allows the palpitation of women students, a most willing form, always with a beatific smile and willingness to remain a passive, pleasuring subject.

Rube is a graduate student in the physics department of the University of Pennsylvania during this time. There are no women in his graduate program. Not much has changed. When I was an undergraduate at Penn in 1941, eight years earlier, I was one of two women in a class of 150 men in the physics course.

As the only married couple in our circle of student friends, Rube and I take advantage of our circumstances and happily arrange several social get-togethers. We have combined picnics in the Wissahickon park and arrange many a *shidach* (match-making).

On many memorable afternoons, we have cookouts, play games, and romp like carefree kids as we relieve our tensions and behave like normal humans instead of serious, humorless, worried students. Some of these new relationships last several years and certainly make the rigors of school more palatable.

The most prominent memories of the past, both fears and pleasures, were made in my first year of medical school, the year of judgment: "To be or not to be."

3

Unexpected Support on the Verge of Disaster

"Copperman, go to Dean Fay's office immediately!"

Thus am I summoned out of class. For what? I can't imagine. My grade scores are fine. My staff relationships are good. I have not cut any classes recently, and I know of no mistakes or harm done to clinic patients. To be pulled out of class this way—I am scared.

"Sit down, Gertrude. I have something serious to discuss with you. I have just now received a call from Dr. Pascal Luchesi to warn me about your activities. He called you a Communist, and he recommends that you be immediately expelled. What is this all about?"

Pulse racing, heart pounding, a familiar frightening choking feeling creeps up into my throat. In a tentative voice, I stammer, "Why, Dr. Fay? Why did he call you? Of what am I guilty?" I grope behind me for the chair and never take my eyes from her face.

I am on a scholarship in my third-year at Woman's Medical College of Pennsylvania. This threat could mean the end of my education and my medical career. To be labeled a Communist in the United States at this time, during the outrageous McCarthy period, is a death knell!

I did have a markedly uncomfortable meeting with Dr. Luchesi last week, but this retribution is unexpected and throws me into a state of panic. He is such a powerful person that his response allows me no recourse. How can I defend myself?

This is the first day back at school after our Christmas holiday, which I had spent at the second annual meeting of AIMS, the national Association of Interns and Medical Students. The meeting was held in the second floor auditorium of the University of Pennsylvania's 100-year-old Houston Hall, a site most significant for me. When I was an undergraduate at Penn in 1943, women were only allowed on the balcony of this building's cafeteria where we sat waiting for our dates to bring lunch up to us. Women were not allowed to enter the cafeteria or any other area of Houston Hall, even though we were fully matriculating university students. Our national meeting last week, well attended by 150 students from all over the United States, was held in this dark, wood paneled, high-ceilinged building that is finally accessible to women.

AIMS's stated goals are to broaden the education of medical students by dealing with social as well as medical issues and to improve the working conditions of interns and residents. Our typical hospital workweek is thirty-four hours on, followed by twelve hours off. At my hospital, an intern's monthly pay is five dollars, just about enough to purchase required stockings.

Our delegates were faced with an unusual problem. Tom, a resident at Philadelphia General Hospital, was discharged from the program because he had a woman in his bedroom on a floor restricted to men. The woman was his wife, but this made no difference.

I was one of five delegates chosen to visit Dr. Luchesi, Philadelphia General Hospital's powerful administrator, to petition for Tom's return to the program. Haughty, scowling, stern, Dr. Luchesi reluctantly granted us an interview. His hostile opening statement set the tone for the brief meeting.

"You have no right to be here," he declared. "This is a city hospital, and Tom knew this was an infraction. The case is closed." Quickly and rudely he escorted us from his office. We couldn't help but wonder if the fact that Tom was trying to organize interns and residents to demand better working conditions hadn't had some influence on Dr. Luchesi's executive decree.

Now quaking in my dean's office, I sit across from a tall, austere, impeccably dressed, white haired woman. Dr. Fay listens without comment as I describe AIMS's program and goals and our meeting with Dr. Luchesi.

When I finish, she says in a heavy Southern accent, "Not only was I called by Dr. Luchesi, but he told me that he has also called the other four schools [of the AIMS delegates] and demanded the other students' expulsions as well."

There is a long silence . . . I cannot imagine what Dr. Fay's response will be. I anxiously await a verdict that could change the entire course of my life. Finally the corners of her lips curl, and a sly smile is just perceptible.

"Gertrude, of course, I will not expel you. Now go back to class. And be careful. There are some dreadful people in our field."

Sweat running down the back of my neck, I must be leaving a damp spot on the bare wooden seat, but I do not look back as I stand. I want to hug her, but in a quavering voice I manage to say, "Thank you, Dr. Fay, for your support and warning." With a sigh of relief and a drop in pulse rate, I hurry back to class.

What a wonderful lady!

Jeep Delivery

1949. My fourth and last year in medical school. Fortunately my scholarship provides most of the required supplies: pens, paper, stethoscope, and otoscope. But I need a means of transportation. As a penniless student, I choose a stripped down Army jeep that costs $150.

My brother David, my greatest advocate and supporter, loans me the money and drives me to an Army surplus depot on the top of a high hill in New Jersey. My purchase made, I clamber up to the high floor—there's no running board. This vehicle is obviously made for a six-footer. I'm five feet and one-half inch tall.

I roar off with David, white-faced, following closely behind me. I fly down a winding, treacherously steep hill. I feel like the jeep has a will of its own. No window flaps, no shock absorbers, no muffler—the roof is a loose-fitting flapping canvas. Wind fills the roof like a balloon and threatens to lift the jeep off the road. I fear it will fly off any moment and soar straight up like a helicopter. Remarkably, the jeep and I make the forty-mile trip back home to Philadelphia safely.

We senior students are required to have our own vehicles for two purposes. One is to transport us around the city to perform home deliveries, of which we each have a quota of babies to fill. The second is to carry maternity patients to local cooperating hospitals when our hospital's newborn nurseries are closed because of infection, in these days before antibiotics. Private patients are told to go to an alternative hospital but not so clinic patients. They present in active labor, ready to deliver, and must be transported rapidly to a nearby cooperating hospital.

My first home delivery is my first procedure without a proctor at my side, the first time I must take full responsibility for two lives, mother and newborn. My companion, Judy, is a fourth-year fellow student. We start out on our first call. It is in the ghetto.

"I'm really excited, Judy. Our first time on our own. We have finally reached medical maturity, but I'm scared shitless. I really feel so much more comfortable with you as my partner, however."

"I'm more scared about this wild ride. I can't believe that we'll get there safely, and in time," Judy responds breathlessly.

"No worry, Judy. You've driven with me through snowstorms and rainstorms. This is a trusty jeep!"

More cautious and traditional in dress as well as outlook than I, Judy has initially trained as a nurse, which makes her the perfect companion. But she's a bit stuffy, as some nurses tend to be.

By this, my last year of formal training, I am feeling confident. Not cocky, but competent to do the job. (At least as I think back, this must have been how I felt or else how could I have survived? This is also before the days of malpractice litigation, which would have certainly induced a feeling of terror. The many possible unforeseen, scary outcomes were only to be realized later, after years in medical practice. Many more than I knew as a novitiate.)

We perform home deliveries in the poorest, most wretched rooms in Philadelphia's ghettos. The neighborhood is strewn with garbage. Trash is piled high on pavements and streets. Roaches and mice scurry away at the sound of our footsteps. Every visit is increasingly distressing.

"Judy, how can people live and children survive in these conditions?"

We arrive at the patient's home noisily because my jeep has no muffler. We unload supplies that are stacked on the floor and back seat of the open jeep. We bring medical equipment and piles of newspapers—paper for cleanliness and sheeting to protect the bed to soak up the blood and amniotic fluid.

I spread the newspaper and whisper so that the laboring mother cannot hear: "Judy, ink is coming off on my hands. What the hell kind of sterility is this?"

"Take it easy, Gert. We have no choice. This is what we have to work with. It's better than the filthy mattress," she whispers.

The mother wears a scanty nightshirt that scarcely covers her huge abdomen. She is lying on a grayish, worn, but seemingly clean sheet that covers only part of the surface of a stained mattress. Stuffing tufts pop out at the seams.

She moans softly at each contraction. This is not her first child. The head is not yet crowning, so we have time to prepare. Inadequately equipped, we have only gloves, suture material for the episiotomy, aspirator for the newborn, and packing material to stanch any abnormal bleeding, but no other prophylactic or emergency materials. (Thinking back today, how could I not have been worried? Suppose it had been a breech that required forceps which we didn't have? We would never have gotten the mother to the hospital in time to save her and the baby. I don't remember considering these possible calamities at the time, however.)

Deliveries, we are taught, most often occur without complications. Luckily this little boy is delivered uneventfully shortly after our arrival.

"A beautiful little brother, Mother," I tell her as I show her the newborn.

We clean the muck, rinse his eyes, and determine that all his parts are present and normal and there's no apparent jaundice. We wrap him in a tattered but clean piece of worn flannel and lay him on his mother's chest. The placenta delivered. There's no excessive bleeding, and we clean up and prepare to leave. (I shudder when I recall and relive these experiences. How did we have the chutzpah to deliver a newborn without adequate help left behind? I don't remember, either, worrying about complications—postpartum hemorrhage, detached placenta, fetal distress. I feel anxious now as I think of all the horrible accidents that could have happened. How lucky, no hemorrhage, no severe jaundice in the newborn requiring hospitalization. How could all of my experiences been free of complications? Or was follow-up so poor in those days? I was not yet a mother myself then and was not fully aware of the help needed for mother and newborn. How inadequate it was to leave a newborn washed down, wrapped in a blanket in mother's arms, and walk off, leaving them alone.)

Someone else must be in the house, but I do not hear any sounds. No one answers my call. Sensing our reluctance to leave her alone, the mother reassures us, "Somebody will be here soon to help me."

Judy and I are distressed at these dreadful living conditions, but fortunately we are not fearful of personal harm in the ghetto. We are certainly an odd couple as we make our rounds in white coats with medical paraphernalia plainly visible in my open, noisy, bare-bones jeep. The sight of us evokes interesting comments from the neighbors. Recognizing us after a few visits to their neighborhood, they call out with waves and smiles, "How are you ladies today? Any new babies?"

My jeep is a remarkable and dependable vehicle, a tough four-wheel-drive and particularly great in the snow. We can push cars up hills when they're stuck on ice or snow. Inclement weather is never a deterrent. The ride is cold, but we always get to our meetings—sometimes eight of us holding on for dear life, our hair and stethoscopes flying in the wind. My classmates' fancy cars might not make it, but we can always pile into my trusty jeep.

It is a lovely, warm spring day, however, when we take a hair-raising jeep ride. The hospital newborn nursery is under quarantine because of a virulent outbreak of the dreaded infectious diarrhea. At this time we have no suitable medications. The only treatment is supportive and isolation. Clinic patients arrive at our hospital in active labor and have to be transported quickly to the Women's Hospital in West Philadelphia, a half-hour away.

I am on duty for the next delivery. When we take off in the jeep, my clinic patient is understandably frightened at this odd means of transportation. But her contractions are a safe twenty minutes apart so I feel confident that we have plenty of time to make the transfer before she goes into hard labor.

We are totally exposed to the streets because the jeep lacks windows and canvas drops. It also has no shock absorbers. My assistant is a third-year medical student, supplied with towels and blankets. She supports our pregnant patient in the back seat and speaks soothingly to her on this windy, unexpected terror-inducing ride.

When we reach the Philadelphia Zoo at 34th Street and Girard Avenue, the hospital is still fifteen minutes away. I suddenly realize that I have not calculated in my jeep's contribution to the woman's labor. I panic. Sans shock absorbers, the bouncing ride produces contractions every five minutes. I anticipate delivery in the back seat of the open jeep.

The expectant mother is now lying down on the back seat and grunting intermittently, crying softly, anxious, and feeling pressure on her perineum. The third-year student continues to talk to her quietly, calming her between contractions, gently massaging her legs, but keeping them squeezed together, hopefully to prevent exodus of the newborn.

I drive like a maniac, one hand on the horn, and pray for a police response, a possible escort, which does not materialize. When we reach the emergency room of the hospital, the contractions are one and a half minutes apart. The bouncing of the jeep is fortunately counteracted by the cooperation of the newborn. His presentation awaits our arrival!

We reach the delivery suite in time for Mom to deliver a beautiful, healthy boy. The trip takes ten years off my life. A jeep proves more effective, I discover, than Pitocin to hasten delivery.

5

Blood, Guts, and Fear

After two years of sitting in lecture halls and dissecting cadavers in labs, I can finally examine my first live person in the third year of medical school, on clinic service. With sweaty hands, I place a stethoscope on a warm body, a live heaving chest. This experience in a supervised, protected environment is my prelude to a life of unremitting tension and insomnia.

Training in our all-female medical school is equal to the best, but hardly preparation for the prejudices of the world awaiting a woman in 1949 when only 11 percent of the practicing medical professionals in the United States were women. Coed medical schools admit women as only 6 percent of their classes. Percentage-wise, there were more female doctors in the United States in 1890 than at the date of my graduation sixty years later. In Philadelphia, there are no female surgeons and many specialties are closed to us.

The only psychiatry course in our curriculum is taught by a father of six who refers proudly to his wife as a *hausfrau*. In one lecture he declares, "Women in professions, especially medicine, are there solely because of penis envy."

What a bastard! We are incensed at his attitude but remain fearfully silent, unlike the outspoken students of today. Growing up as a tomboy, I felt no gender prejudice. Yet my M.D., eight years in the achieving, holds questionable promise in the hostile world he represents.

I am the first woman in ten years to be accepted at Philadelphia's Mt. Sinai Hospital for a one-year rotating internship required by the state. This internship involves one month's service in each specialty and is designed to provide an introduction to the different areas we might specialize in.

My introduction to the hospital staff and my fellow interns and residents is unsettling. I am the only female present. After announcing my name in turn, I remain silent and listen to the easy banter of the all-male audience, many of them already familiar to each other. Is this a preview of a year of feeling odd man out? I wonder. They are talking among themselves like old buddies, as they mostly are, about Saturday night social get-togethers with their wives. I am not included. I sit silently, anxious awaiting the announcements of schedules and duties. The boys seem to be without apprehension. The chief of medicine finally arrives to discuss our rotations, duties, and hours. We then immediately set to work.

On obstetrics service we deliver babies, usually of clinic patients but sometimes private patients if their private obstetrician arrives later than the newborn. Pediatrics is a very noisy clinic where diagnosis and treatment are more difficult because of our young, inarticulate patients. In pathology we learn to conduct post-mortems and have the horrific task of requesting the family's permission for the procedure. Explaining the necessity for autopsy to shocked, grieving, distraught relatives is always a macabre scene, at least for me. My male colleagues appear to be either more detached or better able to hide their feelings.

Emergency room is my first rotation—the roughest, most challenging and frightening service of the year. This ER bears no resemblance to the pristine ERs portrayed on television. Dingy, peeling porcelain cabinets with glass doors hold bandages, scissors, splints, oxygen tanks, aspirating tubes, all manner of emergency equipment and other murderous looking material. Am I supposed to know how to use all this strange paraphernalia?

ERs of the 1950s functioned differently than those of today. Changes began in the 1970s as a result of the drug terror hitting Philadelphia and other cities. Doctors were attacked and murdered in their offices. One-half mile from my home office, a doctor and an armed plainclothes hired guard in his waiting room were both murdered, presumably for drugs. Inner city doctors abandoned their offices. Streets were not safe for women alone in many neighborhoods. One of my elderly patients was attacked shortly after walking out of my office in a comfortable middle-class neighborhood and suffered a fractured skull. When I made house calls at night, I would request an escort to my car in the large parking lots of apartment buildings. I had to close my home office and move into an office building for safety.

The loss of community physicians, terrorized by the violence, then forced patients to use the ERs for general medical care—for fevers, sore throats, and belly aches—not just for emergencies. By contrast, ERs in my day mainly treated severe, often terrible, mutilating, life threatening emergencies.

Mt. Sinai, the hospital where I intern in 1950, is located in South Philadelphia. It serves a community of lower-income working class patients as well as the homeless and families on welfare. Patients arrive seriously ill and require fast responses. I break out into a sweat and palpitations with every arrival.

The ER has one doctor—me—one nurse, and one orderly to take care of all the drunks and sterno-drinking, belligerent patients. We have no beepers so we can only reach the seasoned staff covering us for advice and help by telephone. Duty is thirty-six hours on, twelve off. I am chronically sleep-deprived, but my anxiety keeps me revved up.

We have no ambulance service. Cops bring in emergency calls in their menacing "black Marias," as patrol cars are called by the community that hates them. The police are okay, most of the time, except with rape victims whom they brusquely and rudely cart off to Philadelphia General Hospital. These victims reputedly receive such horrendous treatment that many rapes go unreported. Child rape victims, some as young as two-years-old, are treated with greater consideration at Jefferson Hospital in Center City.

Life in the ER is never dull. For any staff person who happened to be free, it is an exciting place to hang out so I always have company, especially at night when the rest of the hospital is asleep. Herb, a recently graduated resident, often shows up in the ER after work because he misses the excitement. One night Herb answers an emergency call instead of the cops. He finds a knife wound victim lying on a sidewalk. Herb puts the man, whose intestines spill out onto his abdominal wall, into the back seat of his car and drives him to our ER. Luckily he is not hemorrhaging, but blood seeps slowly from the hole in his belly. Despite his guts being splayed out, clean as a surgical dissection, he is still conscious—and terrified.

As we wrap his exposed abdominal organs in saline-soaked towels, we are astonished that there has been no organ perforation. We run him up on the litter to the OR, gently stuff his intestines back in, and sew him up. He walks out well and hearty in five days, only to be returned DOA a week later from a gunshot wound inflicted by his girlfriend's jilted lover.

Terrible, frightening cases always seem to happen in the middle of the night when it is hard to get medical staff backup. At 3 A.M. one winter, the police bring in an unconscious, stinking, filthy, aged man whom they retrieved from the local dump. When they present him to me, he is covered with garbage. The pockets of his tattered pants provide no clues to his identity—only a few scraps of paper, dirty rags, and cardboard to line the soles of his shoes.

This is the worst scenario—a comatose, shallow-breathing patient who requires immediate, life-saving intervention. I shudder as I begin my examination. I am repelled by his foul-smelling breath, but it is without a hint of alcohol. Under his vermin-infested clothing, his skin is layered with dirt and garbage, and his scalp is scabrous and crusting. He must have burrowed under the filth to keep warm. His scrofulous, peeling skin is too dry and too heavily crusted to be adequately cleaned for proper examination.

In the 1950s we do not have the precious laboratory tests or modern equipment to aid in diagnosis that we have today. The first step in this patient's diagnosis is catheterization of the penis to rule out diabetic coma and renal failure. Four male interns are lolling around the ER, looking for excitement because their floor patients are asleep. They approach me separately, not within earshot of the others.

"Gert, let me do the cath for you."

They each think this might be too uncomfortable for a female to perform, especially in a putrid, filthy patient. Terrified, but realizing he might die if I do not act quickly, I thank them, but I know I must do it myself to demonstrate competency and a sense of belonging.

The patient lives long enough to be transported to the OR where we clean up his body and discover large areas of foul smelling necrotic tissue. The surgeon digs fistfuls of dead, rotting remains from both buttocks and finds little viable tissue underneath. Overwhelmed by the awful stench, I want to vomit into my surgical mask. But I hold on as I assist the surgeon because I again hope to prove that I belong in this intern fraternity. The patient cannot be saved, and the suite is closed for twenty-four hours for cleaning and fumigation.

My first surgical "scrub-in" is a simple appendectomy. The surgeon plans to allow me the final cut for removal of the organ. The patient is prepped. His torso is covered with a white sheet, leaving his shaved pelvic area exposed. I approach the table to find laid out on the top of the sheet the largest uncircumcised penis I have ever seen.

"Oh, my," I blurt out. Fortunately the patient is already under but the nurses and Vic, the surgeon, never forgot.

"Any new measurements, Gert?" dogs me for the year.

In fifty years of medical practice, I never find a more cooperative, supportive, congenial, and respectful group than the intern and resident group of that first year. We help each other in many ways.

Blood is drawn from hospital patients at 6 A.M. No technician venipuncture teams in those days. My male colleagues often call upon me when a tough venipuncture stick requires a soft female touch. When the occasional male patient, conscious and often elderly, refuses to allow me to catheterize him, they take over.

Late one night near the end of that year, I am on the private medical floor—the easiest rotation—when four carloads of high school students arrive in the emergency room. They have been in a tragic multi-car accident while returning home from a school basketball game. Several of the youngsters have suffered potentially paralyzing or life-threatening neck injuries. Others have fractures, head injuries, or internal bleeding that require immediate attention. Every intern and resident is summoned off the floors to the emergency room, which leaves me to provide care for the rest of the entire hospital. Fortunately, late at night, most of the patients are asleep.

But emergencies always proliferate. An emergency admission comes in on my hospital floor with bleeding esophageal varices, which are blood vessels at the end of the esophagus where it meets the stomach that have no surrounding muscular bands to contract these abnormally swollen vessels. Esophageal varices, a frequent result of alcoholism and a prominent cause of death in such patients, require immediate surgical intervention. But first the hemorrhaging has to be controlled to survive surgery. We have no suitable equipment available.

Vic is called in to see the patient. A creative surgeon, Vic thinks that a firm rubber catheter (a hollow tube of narrow diameter) could be surrounded by some sort of inflatable material like a narrow balloon to encase the catheter, which could then be introduced into the esophagus. Once in place, it could be inflated to compress the blood vessels and stop the bleeding. A narrow balloon-like material could work, but where could we get it? And quickly?

"Condoms," Vic calls out. "We'll use condoms."

Where to find them at two o'clock in the morning?

"Gert, you're the only free person available," he says as he starts to take the patient to the OR. "Go down and collect them from the guys in the ER."

An unusual request. How will I explain this to the guys who are busy saving lives? When I arrive at the ER, I find a wild, hectic scene. I walk in and announce, "No joking. Vic has sent me down to collect your condoms. He needs them to rig up a device for some emergency surgical intervention."

"Come off it, Gert. You've got to be joking."

"Honest. He has a guy with bleeding esophageal varices, and he has an idea for a device to stop the hemorrhage."

"OK, but you have to dig them out yourself," replies one of the interns with a smirk.

Everyone is gloved to deal with multiple traumas. What to do? Amused by the thought, but realizing I need to act, I have to go into their pants to get their condoms.

"Hey, Gert, what the hell are you doing in my pants?" yells Archie. "Take it easy. You're going in too deep!"

Laughter erupts in this scene of ER mayhem. With no time to explain, I cry, "I need your condoms for Vic."

"Gert, you're a married woman. What are you doing with Vic?" Archie shouts. The others express similar comments as I scurry around the ER to rifle through their pants. I retrieve an amazing colorful collection, which I have to promise to replace.

Vic is able to save the patient's life using those condoms. In a year of scores of sad, funny, and sobering experiences, this is the most memorable episode. Whenever I meet a buddy from those days, we still chuckle at the memory.

We know that condoms save lives—in many different ways. Today, fifty-two years later, physicians use medical equipment called the Blakemore tube that is designed with that condom principle in mind.

That funny, wonderful, frightening year was the greatest preparation for the following fifty. I started fearful and left confident. Remembering it now, I see it as the year in which I reached maturity.

6

Calamity Doc

The internship year ends in June. I am still an unlicensed physician until state examinations are taken and passed in September. An unlicensed physician in this interim period has few employment opportunities. Many of us take jobs at overnight summer camps, as I am now doing. For emergencies and prescriptions I'm covered by local physicians who have been contracted by the camp.

This should be a cushy job—treating colds, sore throats, sunburn, head lice, poison ivy, and bellyaches (usually caused by homesickness)—but it turns into a series of nightmares. Never before or since have I heard reports of camp emergencies like those of my summer of 1950.

At 11:30 the night before camp is to open and the kids arrive, I am called to the bedside of a junior counselor in the boys camp. Bob is scrunched frog-like with his knees pulled up to his chest. He is groaning and trying not to cry.

"Are you a doctor?" he frowns suspiciously. I look younger than my age and he has probably never met a lady doctor.

"Yes, I am. Tell me what's wrong. Where do you hurt?"

"I have a really bad stomachache," he grunts, rolling slowly and painfully on to his back to see me better. He looks frightened. Is it the pain or seeing me?

"How long have you have been hurting?"

"It started after lunch, but now it's really awful," he groans louder. His only exposed area, his hairless, boyish face, is pale, panic stricken, and drenched in sweat. He is hot under bed covers that he holds protectively up to his chin. Is this seventeen-year-old youngster even going to allow me to touch him?

"Have you had any vomiting or diarrhea? Have you ever had anything like this before?"

"No," he answers distrustfully.

"I'm going to examine you and will try not to hurt you."

Tugging at the covers, he quickly pulls the sheet up over each area of naked torso after I finish palpating it. My gauge of anxiety, my armpits, are already wet. Could this be acute appendicitis, needing immediate action? But his tenderness and muscle guarding are in the right upper quadrant under the liver, not in the right lower quadrant, at McBurney's point, the usual place for a hot appendix. Could this be the unusual subhepatic appendix that I have read about but never seen? Unlikely to be gall bladder disease in a seventeen-year-old. His liver is not enlarged, and there is no radiation of pain to his back.

I am anxious. I try not to show it, but in a quavering voice, I explain, "You will have to be taken to the hospital, Bob. I think this is appendicitis."

"Oh, no. Camp starts tomorrow!"

"I'm sure you will be on your feet and back in camp in a week, but you really have no choice but to go." I try patting his shoulder comfortingly, but under the covers he cringes and shrinks at my touch. "I'll call your parents now and get you admitted. I will put you on the phone so that you can talk to them."

The covering doc at the closest hospital fortunately accepts my diagnosis and its urgency. He arranges the admission just on my description. To save time, he agrees to meet us at the hospital. We don't wait for an ambulance, which could mean a half-hour delay. Bob is bundled into the back seat of the camp car. He is cold, though his shivering body is covered by a pile of blankets. He softly sobs as I speed along a narrow, poorly lit country road.

Within the hour Bob is operated on, even before his parents can arrive. A hot appendix in an unusual location! We do get to it before it ruptures. We are both lucky and greatly relieved. Bob's recovery is prompt, and he returns to camp in a week. He recovers faster than my apprehension for the summer ahead.

   The next several weeks are calm and quiet. I enjoy the kids and staff. I always have ready tennis partners, great swimming weather, and lots of free time. But after questions from some of the campers, I feel compelled to address certain key issues, such as personal relations, sexual changes, and their impact in the different age groups. After somewhat reluctant permission from the bosses, I am allowed to meet with different age groups weekly. Attendance is good, especially in the older age groups. This is a new experience for most of us. I have never tried anything like this and, to add to my discomfort, several of the participants are my senior. After some early hesitation to talk, we all loosen up a bit.

   With the ten-year-olds I start discussing menses, its significance in body development, and the use of Tampax. In 1950 many have never seen or heard of Tampax. Following my discussion with this age group, their counselor corners me on the hilltop, alone.

   "I strongly disagree with you. I object to your talk with these younger kids. I think it's the mothers' job to discuss menses and especially the use of Tampax with their daughters. I feel you are overstepping your boundaries." She is very angry, but after some discussion we end up amicably. Interesting outcome: This counselor not only becomes my patient but she also brings her mother and sister as patients when I open my first office. Many of the folks I meet at camp subsequently become my patients as well, which is very gratifying.

   The older age group, which includes Morris the camp director, is a bit daunting for me. We discuss personal relations, sex, and prophylaxis. Some of the questions are amazing and frightening in display of their ignorance.

   "When is the woman's safe period, to be able have sex without protection against pregnancy?" [This was long before HIV.] They are surprised and disbelieving at my response: "There is no such time because one never knows in advance when one's cycle and ovulation time may change." This answer takes a lot of convincing and drawing of diagrams.

"Am I safe if he withdraws before ejaculation?" It is hard to convince them of the facts, especially because the young males object to my response of "No way."

The summer finally evolves into what it was supposed to have been until an incident occurs that ends my anxiety-free days and restful nights.

The camp director's wife is a "drone," as camp mates are called. Eight of her pregnancies had ended in early spontaneous abortions. Their only living child, Anna, is a brittle juvenile diabetic, easily prone to illnesses and infections with just minor trauma.

I am awakened from sleep by Betty, Anna's frightened bunk counselor.

"Come quickly. Anna is breathing funny and has a terrible bellyache!"

I grab a jacket and as we run to her bunk, Betty, scared and breathless, fills me in. "She was fine at lights-out but woke just now crying and complaining of her belly."

"Run and get Morris while I see her."

Anna is lying in a pool of sweat, shivering, ashen gray, with acetone breath. She is able to be aroused but is surely sinking into diabetic acidosis. I find right lower quadrant tenderness this time. My second emergency appendicitis in one summer—I want to go home!

We race to the closest hospital. I'm still in pajamas. Unprofessional attire, particularly in a hospital run by nuns. We enter an austere, gray-walled corridor unrelieved by any adornment except for pictures of a tortured Christ on the cross. The nuns are a fearsome sight, black raiment sweeping the floor, heads bound revealing only foreheads, noses, and mouths. Are we are entering a medieval cloister, I wonder.

Anna luckily receives immediate attention. Surgery is performed stat, fortunately before rupture. Diabetes controlled, she returns to camp in one week. She is a spunky kid. In later years I have many anxious episodes with Anna. She would die at the age of twenty-eight, the first death in my practice.

I no longer expect the usual camp norm, but I am totally unprepared for the next calamity. One week before the end of the season, I am awakened by a strange whirring sound. My entire bedspread, the walls and the ceiling of the bunk, are covered with black crawlies. I flee in my pajamas. Lucky I did not sleep in the buff that night. I never did find the source or name of the invaders. My clothes are debugged and later delivered to me, but I never do return to that bed.

A fitting end to an unusual summer job.

7

Cost Effective Lives

"If you do not put your finger into your patient's butt yearly, you will one day put your foot in it," warns every clinical professor of physical examination at medical school.

Approximately 70 percent of all colon cancers, they claim, are within reach of the examining finger, i.e. within the first four inches of the anus. Feces withdrawn on the doctor's gloved finger can also be examined for the presence of blood. This "hemoccult test" can potentially demonstrate the presence of malignant polyps that are asymptomatic at this time, out of reach of the examining finger and further up in the intestinal tract. The manual examination also evaluates the prostate gland and potential pathology in female genital organs.

"You perform more rectal hemoccult examinations than any other GP within a 250-mile radius," scolds the critical and threatening Blue Cross/ Blue Shield representative on his yearly visit to my office in the early 1970s. "I am again advised to warn you that this test is not considered cost-effective, and your request for repayment will soon be censured."

He is a short, unsmiling ogre in a black suit and tightly knotted tie. I make the same angry assertion every time this evil looking agent visits me. "Tell the other doctors on your route that for the sake of their patients, they should be doing this yearly as well."

His threats, however, leave me anxious, worried, and fearful of what further action his organization might one day take. And they eventually do.

The criticism and threat emanate from the cost-conscious corporate medical directors who provide the cheapest minimal medical services to many thousands of employees. The examinations are part of the service contract for the employees, but there are no legal precedents for what each company provides. They do not consider the hemoccult test cost-effective. They figure it is cheaper to treat a terminal patient who has symptomatic colon cancer than to do simple, cheap tests on thousands of factory workers. Patients reaching the symptomatic stage do not live long. Colon cancer detected in its early stage has a five-year survival rate of 90 percent, while those in the later stage have an 8 percent survival rate.

This hemoccult test is reimbursed for all of $3.50—hardly an excessive payment considering the time involved, the cost of gloves and chemicals, and the time to discuss it with patients before and after the procedure, particularly the occasionally embarrassed resistant ones who are most often males.

During one of those procedures, I startled a patient: "I thought you had given up smoking." The surprised patient twisted his head on the table so that he could look at me, "How could you tell from that end?"

"You have a pipe sticking out of your pocket." I often use this joke to relax my patient.

The insurance companies compensating for office procedures are irate at my refusal to curtail this practice and report me to the appropriate health agencies that control the practice of medicine and its reimbursement in the state of Pennsylvania. I am summoned to Harrisburg to appear before an all-male peer group to defend my activity. Would my honest and cheap valid procedure be condemned? Would I then be fined and required to pay back $3.50 for every patient on whom I had performed this test yearly? This would be hundreds. I have many sleepless nights as I comb my records for supporting documentation.

Over a period of four years, four asymptomatic colon cancers are diagnosed and their removal produces a cure that requires no further treatment. Dr. S., the surgeon to whom I refer patients, writes a letter for me to present to the group asserting the noteworthy results of my procedures and commending me on the nature of my practice.

Fortuitously at this time, the American Cancer Society publishes an article recommending that hemoccult tests be done yearly. I feel supported and reinforced but still scared. Appearing before this inquisitorial assembly alone looms overwhelmingly. I need someone to come with me. I ask my friend and office assistant who, after twenty-five years of working with me, is as close as a sister. "Pauline, I really can't do it alone. Will you drive to Harrisburg with me?"

"I will not only come, I will drive. Working with you for twenty-five years in this office, I wouldn't dare trust you to do the driving when you are so stressed out."

I am terror-stricken at the prospect of facing an all-male peer group who might very well be unaccepting of a woman doctor. At this time, less than 11 percent of practicing physicians in the United States are women. I have attended medical meetings where I am the only woman. I just have to take a deep breath and start talking and all eyes are averted. A sense of ennui descends as the men present doubt my comments are worth hearing.

A typical attitude at one of those meetings: In his presentation of hypertensive disease, the discussant blatantly states, "Women, unlike men, do not develop high blood pressure from workplace stress. They are only out to work because they are bored housewives." After too many of these experiences, I stop attending these discussion groups.

We finally reach Harrisburg and are ushered into the company of six unsmiling males who barely utter a polite greeting. Their formal attire, stern facial expressions, and stiff postures do not indicate a courteous or sympathetic audience. I already feel judged and condemned. I know I am doomed. They read my material. After a very few questions, some addressed to Pauline as well, they caucus.

To my great relief, their appearance is not reflective of their attitude and decision. "Dr. Copperman, your practice is commendable. We agree this should be a regular office procedure." Appearances can certainly be deceiving.

Pauline and I have a victory lunch and a glass of wine. I can only manage the wine.

It would be nice to conclude that money does not control the practice of medicine. Or does it?

That hearing took place in the 1970s. Thirty years later, on November 2, 2001, an important announcement is made on national television. A significant new medical development could change the practice of medicine and reveal early colon pathology as nothing else to date has done. This test was actually known in the 1950s, the one for which I was criticized, and they are describing this as a new discovery. Imagine describing the hemoccult test as something new on the horizon!

Of course they recommend it be done with sensitivity. A cardboard packet is given to the patient to be smeared with feces at home and returned to the doctor or laboratory by mail. This mailed specimen has been reputed to result in false negatives because the dried out material is poorly reconstituted. No manual examination is done that could reveal other multiple pathologies in a woman's genital area and the male's prostate area. It's a shortcut that potentially produces inaccurate results and does not recognize the value of the physical examination. Automated medicine. No need for the physician. Medicine by mail!

8

I Was a Felon

I am twenty years old and pregnant. It's 1942. My husband is shipping out to war. Scarred, trembling, anxious, apprehensive, not knowing what to expect, I am sure that discovery could mean jail for the operating physician and me.

In my first year after college, I am the lowest rung research assistant at The Children's Hospital of Philadelphia and barely able to support myself. How can I support a child? Am I being irresponsible, endangering my life? Will I be able to bear children in the future? Will this person be a doctor? I am aware of women, with no husband and the burden of pregnancy, who choose suicide.

From a heavily trafficked street, I enter a poorly lit hallway that leads to a darkly curtained, dingy waiting room. It is shabbily furnished and smells musty. Hardly a clean or secret location. I want to run. But I have no alternative.

My friend's mother, a nurse in New York City, has arranged this appointment. An esteemed gynecologist initially interviewed me in his well-appointed office to ascertain my emotional stability. A referral from him led to this shabby, unprofessional-looking office on a main thoroughfare in Manhattan. The contrast is unexpected and unnerving.

An assistant enters after a short wait. Her appearance is hardly reassuring. Mousy gray hair, wrinkled spotted uniform. Is it dried blood? Without any introduction, she hands me a plastic container.

"Empty your bladder." I take the container and enter a dim cubicle with peeling wallpaper, a dirty toilet, and grimy sink. It reeks of urine, maybe old blood. After I hand back the container, I am ushered into another room with an examining table equipped with stirrups. There are no IV stands or other medical equipment, just a lamp and cruddy storage cabinets in need of paint.

The doctor is fully masked and capped, unrecognizable except for thick glasses. He begins without addressing me by name and cleans the perineal area without a word. I look up into the face of his gap-toothed assistant as she administers ether, drop by drop into a cone that covers my nose and mouth. The anesthesia is inadequate. I feel each swipe of the curette as it scrapes the inner layer of my uterus.

I'm discharged an hour later, still groggy, with a bellyache but no hemorrhage. Safely out on the street, I feel lucky. I'm alive, and at least I've had a real doctor in New York City. Sixty years later, I still feel the terror and horror of how the abortion was arranged and performed.

In 1945, three years after the abortion, I enter Women's Medical College in Philadelphia. This 150-year-old institution is the only all-female medical college in the world, but we receive only one hour of lecture on birth control during our four years there. The lecture is delivered not by our staff but by a male representative from the Sanger Planned Parenthood Clinic in Philadelphia. Not even a physician, and a male, comes to discuss contraception at an all-female medical school. Catholic students are not allowed to attend the session. The Sanger Clinic, run by physicians not associated with our medical school, is under constant attack by the church and pro-lifers.

The course content at medical institutions at this time is under the control of many non-medical groups. Church and state adjudicate the issue of birth control, not our teaching institutions. In four years at an all-female medical college, we do not hear a single hour of lecture on sex education. These are, in truth, the dark ages.

Prohibitions are such that we are not allowed to discuss contraception with patients in obstetrical and gynecologic clinics. We cannot prescribe methods of protection, even though future pregnancies could be potentially life threatening in some patients.

Our instructors closely monitor us so we can only discuss what is then rigidly controlled.

The Sanger Clinic address is posted on a chalkboard. We quietly point it out to patients: "You need to write down this address. This clinic will provide birth control information."

Secretly a group of us goes to the Sanger Clinic after class, at night, to learn the principles of birth control and the fitting and use of contraceptive diaphragms. Abortions are illegal in the United States except in rare medical circumstances. Laws in some states even control purchases of contraceptive aids. In Massachusetts, for example, contraceptive materials—condoms, diaphragms, and even contraceptive creams—cannot be bought without a doctor's prescription.

We receive no instruction about how or when an abortion is to be performed even for the legally allowed therapeutic procedure. Only gynecologists can perform these surgeries. Our women teachers are mainly conservative. We fear expulsion if our attendance at the clinic is discovered. We swear our classmates to secrecy.

Medical school graduation arrives in 1949. After an internship and residency and the birth of one daughter, I open an office for general medical practice. One of the major problems facing me at this time is the safety of my women patients of child-bearing age. In mid-twentieth century America, the leading cause of death among women ages sixteen to twenty-six is septic abortion. These deaths result from procedures' being performed in secrecy by untrained persons without medical supervision or from self-induced attempts by desperate young women.

These women have only a choice of backroom abortions on kitchen tables in upstate Pennsylvania or self-induced abortions with hat pins or coat hangers that can pierce the cervix, perforate the uterus, and cause infections that can end in death. Old wives' tales of purging, scalding baths, self-mutilation are painful but ineffective.

We physicians are powerless to help. Doctors brave enough or foolhardy enough to perform illegal abortions in their offices are jailed and have licenses revoked in both the United States and

Canada. If and when a hospital board can be convinced of the necessity of the procedure, abortions in the hospital are safe, simple, and have no harmful after effects.

Women who can afford it travel to France or Switzerland where abortion is legal. But this is not always certain. My phone rings at 4 A.M. A patient named Sally, calling from Switzerland, is crying hysterically. With an overseas operator listening in, I have to counsel her.

"I need a letter from a psychiatrist saying that I'm mentally competent to have an abortion," Sally sobs.

I promise to send a letter. For many months thereafter I expect a call from the FBI. I am certain that the operator has reported our conversation.

Many of my patients are dissuaded from using unsafe, drastic means to end unwanted pregnancies. I can call upon agencies like Concerned Clergy for Pregnancy that somehow are able to arrange for abortions through their own secret networks. But unfortunately, these networks operate at some distance from Philadelphia and are not accessible to my poorer patients.

Those patients who can be helped are very loyal and protective. As an intern, I observe a patient who is admitted through the Emergency Room with a perforated uterus and peritonitis, an unusual and lethal complication. Even though she knows she is dying, she refuses to name her doctor. This occurs before the era of effective antibiotics, which might have saved her life. Hounded by police stationed at her door—round the clock in three eight-hour shifts and checking all her visitors—she dies without revealing her surgeon's name.

In the late 1960s, the independent, headstrong daughter of a friend is carrying an unwanted pregnancy. Jane is about to fly to Puerto Rico to a secret, word-of-mouth abortion mill. I am distraught by not having the resources to help her here. Although Jane can afford the expensive excursion, my primary concern is her safety at this unknown clinic. I beg every gynecologist friend I have for help, without success. I am so desperate that I'm close to purchasing simple aspiration equipment and performing the procedure myself.

"Gert, don't do it. You'll surely go to jail. You won't get away with it," my colleagues warn.

Concerned for Jane's safety and frustrated by the lack of help and caring that I encounter, I cannot relax. I take off for the track. Running always calms me and clears my mind. I tend to perseverate when problems seem insolvable, but solutions often come to me when I'm exercising. It happens once again—the solution hits me.

I remember that, during my second year of medical school, I was assigned to write an original paper on a subject of my own choosing. I was interested in genetics and had been intrigued by an article in an Australian medical journal. As I run around the track, I recall that paper on the effect of German measles (Rubella) during the first trimester of pregnancy.

German measles was unknown in Australia until American GIs introduced it to that continent in World War II. When Australian women contracted the disease from American soldiers in their first three months of pregnancy, they had a statistically significant number of congenitally deformed infants. Therapeutic abortion since then is routinely recommended in Australia to infected women. This medical response to German measles is not generally known, nor is it a frequent recommendation in the United States at this time, the 1960s. Physicians who are aware of it are often hampered from acting on the information by their hospital boards.

Could this be the answer? I wonder as I run.

After twenty years of facing this problem and appalled at the many complications, illnesses, and deaths caused by illegal, botched, unprofessionally performed abortions, I finally devise an approach to help my patients. It is a felony, but the passage of time makes me safe from prosecution today.

I use this information over the course of many years to save many women from disastrous outcomes. I claim to diagnose the first trimester of German measles in my patients who are carrying unwanted pregnancies. I never use the same physician twice, never admit to the same hospital where I have previously used this diagnosis, and never refer to a physician or hospital whose religion will not allow abortions to be performed for any reason. Almost to a person, gynecologists accept my fabricated diagnosis and perform this simple, very safe procedure under aseptic conditions in a hospital.

My plan is first threatened when Alice, a trusted patient whom I've known since she was an adolescent, cries piteously, wrings her hands, and paces nervously. She is so distressed that she cannot stay still.

"I'm pregnant. John and I have split," she sobs. "He is back on drugs and I cannot support a third child on my meager income."

Alice is a young struggling artist who works menial jobs. I speak to her obstetrician who had delivered her two children. He agrees to perform the abortion—if.

"Gert, I will perform the blood test for Rubella on Alice in the hospital. If it's negative, the procedure will not be done."

No other doctor has demanded this test. I feel certain that he is bluffing because this new blood test is prohibitively expensive. But I'm scared.

He does, in fact, perform the abortion without the blood test. I guess his threat to me was to cover his butt, or he expected me to back down if my diagnosis was a fabrication. Ironically, the same physician is described in the newspapers the following week as a leading proponent for legalized abortions.

The 1974 Roe V. Wade decision makes abortions legal, but we physicians and patients face severe problems today, despite this legal victory. I believe that it is a woman's right to choose. If she chooses the path of abortion, she should have the right to safe, aseptic conditions as guaranteed by our legal system without the threat of physical attack.

Have our struggles been in vain, I wonder. Will we be felons again?

9

A Tough Call: An Angel On My Shoulder

Pelting sleet, heavy snow, mounting drifts. I imagine the Alaskan tundra, but I am free to walk and enjoy the cold blistering winds that clear my head of the worries and anxieties that are so much a part of my life.

No office hours today. Storms are rough telephone days, though. Patients worry about reaching a doctor in a blizzard. No one dares venture out, so calls flood the office and telephone advice is the treatment of the day. I can call my exchange from home to get messages, but problems are more readily handled with access to patients' charts in my office. This is my excuse I give my daughters for walking through the storm to my office two miles away.

I enjoy this weather, in fact. Not many cars on the road today. A very occasional passing driver, known or unknown to me, offers a ride.

"Thank you for stopping, but I really love walking in the snow." They stare, unbelieving and quizzical. They must think that I'm some kind of nut to refuse their offers, especially those who recognize me as bundled up as I am.

"Come on, Copperman. Get in or you'll catch pneumonia." I smile and wave them on. I rationalize that it is safer to walk than to drive through the drifting, slippery snow covering the roadways.

After plodding nearly two miles along neighborhood side streets, I reach City Line Avenue, the major thoroughfare where my office is located. This four-lane street has no vehicular traffic today. Instead, cross-country skiers claim the road all to themselves. Traffic is almost universally at a standstill throughout the entire city, so I'm surprised to notice several patrons in the beauty salon located in my office building. They've come from several fancy apartment complexes within walking distance.

As soon as I enter my office, the phone rings. I'm still shaking snow off my coat.

"Thank God you're in!" The manager of the beauty salon is breathless and shouting. "Please, Dr. Copperman, you must see my very sick employee. You are the only doctor in the building today. She is vomiting and fainting."

"Get her right in here. My office is Suite 52, intermediate level."

I anxiously await her arrival. Faced with an emergency and an unknown patient, I am as tense as the patient. Despite my years in practice, my pulse is racing, my breathing is labored, and my armpits are wet.

Soon a pale, limp young woman arrives. Mary vomits profusely into a bucket held by one of her supporters. Two other people hold her, one on each side. As they help her in, she can barely walk. I expect her to pass out momentarily.

Mary's supporters appear as frightened as the patient. They aren't the only ones scared. Faced with an unknown woman who's obviously very ill and can scarcely speak, I am afraid, too. Her vomiting is projectile, shooting out uncontrollably and forcefully at a distance. It has a stinking fecal stench.

Projectile vomiting immediately suggests a possible neurologic involvement, a lesion, pathology, or infection in the brain—a scary emergency. Examination provides no clues. She is afebrile, (that is, she has no fever by rectal temperature), no headache, and no abdominal tenderness.

An injection of compazine stops the vomiting as long as she lies flat. But any attempt to sit her up again results in more projectile vomiting. While she reclines, I am able to question Mary. She tells me she'd been using birth control pills properly, has had a recent menses, and has no abdominal pain. This information pretty well rules out a tubal ectopic pregnancy. The neurologic examination is surprisingly negative. Only projectile vomiting continues.

One of her attendants pipes up, "We all had egg salad sandwiches swimming in mayo, but no one else is sick. The manager treated us all to the same lunch since we couldn't get out for lunch because of the storm." But since her co-workers aren't sick, this makes a diagnosis of food poisoning unlikely.

I am worried. I feel that the findings, or lack thereof, warrant hospitalization, but neither Mary nor her mother, who has been contacted by telephone, is easily convinced. I am a stranger to them, and they resent my questions about pregnancy to an unmarried very religious young woman.

My insistence and anxiety finally force their acceptance, and they agree to the hospital admission. As Mary sets off with my blankets, my buckets, and her three attendants, she is still vomiting when upright. They head out into this raging blizzard in an automobile. No ambulance or police can be reached.

Fortunately Larry, my neurologist, is still at the hospital. He agrees to await her arrival despite a certain delay caused by the storm. He knows me well, responds to my anxiety, and trusts my judgment. We are worried as we discuss on the phone the possibility that the hospital might refuse admission because we have no clear diagnosis. (This is before the days of diagnostic CAT scans and MRIs and—luckily—before the days of HMO's and their restrictive cost-containment policies, which dangerously limit hospital admissions.)

They reach the hospital despite the storm and Larry is waiting. Mary's only symptom is still projectile vomiting—but with no further neurologic findings. No fever, no pain, no headache. All we have to go on is a high level of suspicion.

At 3 A.M. that night, Mary suddenly develops a headache and nuchal rigidity, which is a stiffness of the neck—a clear sign of neurologic involvement. A neurosurgeon is called and arrives wet, dripping with snow, but promptly and safe. He operates on Mary's leaking cerebral aneurysm and saves her life.

Larry calls me the next morning, shaken but relieved.

"Gert, had this been July, with the beginning of the rotation of new, inexperienced interns, instead of December, Mary would likely have been sent home with a diagnosis of gastroenteritis, upset stomach. Then she would have been readmitted the next day a DOA."

When he makes that statement, Larry doesn't know that Mary's fianceé had been a DOA three months earlier. The post mortem diagnosis was a ruptured cerebral aneurysm. A remarkable coincidence!

10

Sexism: Second Class Women

In the early 1970s a psychiatrist named Karl is treating one of my patients. In fact, Martha and her whole family are my patients. At some point in therapy, Karl asks me to join him in conducting several family sessions because he believes it will help Martha, her siblings, and their spouses. Initially Martha is most resistant because she prefers to keep control by hanging on to her illness. Several joint sessions, however, seem to help the entire family. This success then prompts Karl to ask for my intervention with a group of somewhat desperate freshmen students—all women—in his class at a local medical school.

"Gert, come to dinner and I'll invite these women over to meet you afterward. I think that your experiences coming through medical school at a time that was even less receptive to women could be helpful to them. I'm sure you've met the same difficulties, and worse, during your time in med school. These women don't know any female physicians so I think it would be good for them to meet a woman doc who's out in practice."

"I'd be delighted to come. You don't have to bribe me with dinner, but that would be nice." I've heard that Karl is a superb cook, and I've never been served a dinner totally prepared by a man except in a restaurant. That evening, in his partially rehabbed Victorian mansion in Germantown, I enjoy turnips like I've never tasted before. I can't wheedle the recipe out of him. The whole meal was a delicious new experience.

One of the freshmen students rents a room in Karl's capacious house, so he is aware of their distress and has become a confidant of several women in his class. During dinner I ask Karl, "What would you like me to discuss with them? Anything special?"

"Just wait 'til they start, Gert. You'll hear a litany of complaints."

After dinner five young women arrive together. I am happy to see Diane who had been a best friend of my daughter Joan in high school. The most comfortable of the group, Diane starts the discussion: "Gert, you would not believe what we face every day from these bigoted, sexist men." Her voice quavers. She's near tears.

"Tell me more about it. And don't forget that I went to an all-female medical school. Some of our professors were sexists, but basically I didn't face your environment until I graduated."

The other four women sit quietly, unsmiling. Perhaps they're uncomfortable in Karl's presence even though they trust him and obviously find him sympathetic.

"I remember your stories," Diane says. "But what's happening to us is more than we expected. We don't even have any restrooms for women in the medical school building."

"I really can't stand the daily insults anymore," says Ruth, whose scowl makes her seem the angriest of the group. "I just don't go to some of the classes. I send my recording machine instead."

"What kinds of insults?" I ask. "Are you personally attacked? What's going on?"

"When we stand up to object to a slur, the boys respond in a single voice: 'Oh, shut up, already,' or they boo."

"Like what slurs?"

"Well, for instance, when the radiologist puts a woman's chest x-ray on the screen, he refers to her breasts as two fried eggs. The guys all guffaw. They shout us down as being 'too sensitive' when we object. Or they yell, 'Can't you take a joke?'"

"These insults may seem insignificant," Diane adds. "But when these sexy slurs are made in every possible instance, the whole day becomes unbearable. They treat us, our bodies, as inferior. We feel ridiculed and insulted in every so-called humorous instance."

Sally, who has been sitting quietly, joins in. "A professor pulled down the screen showing the body of a nude woman the other day. Using his pointer, he applied too much pressure over the *mons pubis* and it caused the screen to roll up. Then he says, 'That's the first one that ever jumped away from me.' That really brought the house down."

"What have you women tried to do in response?" I ask.

"We're such a small group in this huge class of men. We appealed to the dean to ask that a woman counselor be assigned to us. His response was, 'There already is a student counselor, and he is adequate to respond to all the students, male and female.' That ended the discussion."

This encounter disturbs me as well as these young students. So little has changed over the past two decades since I was in medical school. Relating statistics about more women entering medicine today, compared to my time, does little to assuage the distress of these 1970s women. They have yet to meet their first female doctor in medical school. I think they feel better after airing their complaints and frustration, but I want to give them more.

I tell them about AIMS (the Association of Interns and Medical Students) that works to affect changes in medical education. But they are at first hesitant. Many students who join and work with such a militant group anticipate retribution and live in fear of being flunked out of school for political reasons, especially in medical schools that are as reactionary as this one.

I remind them that the first woman to go through medical school in New York City had to masquerade as a man and never revealed her identity until graduation. I also point out that the AMA didn't admit women or African Americans as members until 1920. A prestigious, 150-year-old medical school in Philadelphia never admitted African Americans until the Army sent them as part of a group during World War II. The school had to accept them then. The same medical school did not admit women until 1965.

"These historic facts don't make your struggles any easier," I tell the women sitting and listening in Karl's living room, "but you have no alternative except to band together. Find those people on the faculty, like Karl, to help sensitize your classmates. It is also important to be aware that we have made many positive changes."

I hope they feel better after this evening, but I know that chances for immediate change are *de minimus*. After tea and cookies, we leave Karl's home somewhat comforted as a group but knowing that the future is still going to be a struggle for a woman doctor.

11

Globalization of Giardia

My patient, Joann, is an artist, a graduate of an elite academy who lives an alternative lifestyle in an ungentrified neighborhood adjacent to a South Philadelphia ghetto. She enjoys pot and probably other so-called social drugs. I worry about communicable diseases whenever she visits my office. In the 1970s, I anticipate anything and everything unusual, but her situation is beyond any expectation.

"I've had terrible cramps and bouts of really violent, almost uncontrollable diarrhea lasting for two to three days," Joann tells me. "Then it disappears and comes back in a few weeks. Nothing seems to help while I have it, and nothing prevents it from reoccurring. Paregoric and kaopectate help a little, but it still lasts about three days and keeps coming back."

I don't ask her where she got the paregoric without a prescription.

"I've had this now about three or four months." Her whining and frowning show she's irritated and wants to blame someone or something.

"Have you changed your diet in any way?"

"No. It doesn't seem related to what I eat or alcohol or anything else. I can't pinpoint it. I went to Mexico years ago and got *tourista* then, but it eventually went away. This has going on for months."

"You haven't been out of this country recently, have you?"

"No, and as far as I know, I haven't eaten at any questionable restaurants, or crazy raw foods."

"Have you eaten *steak tartare* or anything that could have been contaminated, like raw fish?"

"Not so far as I can remember," she replies with a grimace. She seems impatient with my questioning.

"Well, I'd better culture your stool. I will call you as soon as I get a result. In the meantime, stay on a bland diet, and I will give you some medicine for the diarrhea in case it recurs before I get the lab results. Take this container and try now to give me a specimen."

"I'll try, but I don't know if I can produce on command now."

"That's okay. Take the container with you and return it soon after the specimen is obtained. What I've ordered for you will keep you comfortable until we get the results."

Unsmiling and annoyed at not receiving an instant cure, Joann takes the container and returns it three days later. To my surprise, her stool cultures out *Giardia*, a rare disease in the United States. The first and last time I've heard of this intestinal parasite was twenty years ago in a lecture on infectious diseases. I am sure that treatment must have changed in the interim. I call the Board of Health to report this communicable disease and to find out the latest treatment. The technician is as surprised as I am. His first response is a question: "What, you have a case of *Giardia*? Has your patient been to the Soviet Union?" Is he suggesting this is a communist spread disease?

"Why? She hasn't been out of the country at all recently. Why the Soviet Union?"

"The only case reports we have on record are those of a tour group recently returned from Leningrad and Moscow wherein we discovered that *Giardia* is endemic in the drinking water supply of both cities. Yours is the first case I have on record other than this group."

This is shocking news. Joann denies any contact with this group. We never can trace the source of her infection. None of her known associates report any illness. At this time, hers and the Russian tourists are the only reported cases in the city. Joann responds well to medication, which I myself at a later date unfortunately do not.

On a trip to Guatemala in the 1980s, I suffer a most distressing, uncomfortable, and intimate exposure. This trip is arranged by my friends, Carole and Chris, who are sports psychologists on staff at Temple University and two of the national organizers of U.S. Women's Sports Foundation. They are attempting to extend this organization to include women in Central and South America. Guatemala is to be the first site of the international meeting.

The sixteen women in our travel group come from all over the United States and represent several fields in sports, education, and health. I am invited to join a panel on the topic of "Exercise for good health in the *Troisieme Etage*," as the third stage or the age group 60 and older, is called in Guatemala. I am to discuss the physiology and the health benefits of exercise and to demonstrate the procedures.

For me, it's a blast. Not only to leave the pressures of practice for eight days but also to be part of a program that I feel is so important in the pursuit of good health—regular exercise at every age. In the 1980s, sports for women is just on the upswing in the United States.

We receive a magnificent welcome in Guatemala. We are housed in a swank hotel, but we're soon horrified by the living conditions, the poverty, and the overwhelming military presence we see in the streets. Soldiers with rifles stand at every corner. They are in the doorways of every store, not just the banks, but at restaurants and parks as well. They are present from early morning to late at night. We don't feel safe. We feel threatened and frightened at the dreadful conditions in this poverty stricken, heavily armed country.

The hotel atmosphere, however, is congenial and safe, and the meetings are freely attended, mainly by middle-class, educated youngsters and women. Cautiously we drink only boiled water, without ice cubes, even though this is summer and extremely hot. We eat all our meals in the hotel—only cooked foods, no salads or fresh fruit. Our single exception: one meal in a pizza parlor. We foolishly decide that this cooked food would be safe. A grave error. The second week after my return home, I develop sudden volcanic bouts of diarrhea. It cultures out *Giardia* and is totally unresponsive to all known medications. Mine is the first case that my gastroenterologist had seen. Every three to four weeks the cysts erupt suddenly from their abodes clustered on my intestinal wall and discharge their contents into my gut.

At one point in the middle of a tennis game with my daughter Joan, I have to lie down on the grass. Joan is sure I am terminal. I've never been known to walk off a court while playing with my kids. After about a year and a half, the invaders finally give out or give up, and I thankfully regain my energy.

With increased foreign travel of Americans and increased emigrations from Central and South America since the 1980s, this organism has invaded mountain streams and lakes throughout the United States. This development, however, is not generally known. When we arrive at a Massachusetts campground in the 1990s, we are surprised to be greeted by a forest ranger warning: "Do not drink the water unless you have the special filter to remove *Giardia*."

The same summer a friend and his three grandsons, who played in the shallow waters of Lake Wallenpaupack in Pennsylvania's Pocono Mountains, all come home with *Giardia* in their intestines. These parasites can now be found in the waterways throughout the United States. In just twenty years, these intestinal grippers have become a global phenomenon.

12

The Perilous Course of a Sick Doctor

Cancer, the dreaded diagnosis. I've always been healthy. I exercise daily, eat well, enjoy my work. No more than the usual stress. Why me? There must be some mistake.

I've had a soreness inside my cheek for about a year. The dentist checks it regularly and believes it's a benign lesion, but it's too far back for me to be able to see. It's always tender whenever my tongue locates the area, which occurs daily, of course.

I know that I have *mitral valve prolapse* (MVP), which means that a valve in my heart is somewhat thicker than usual and billows (or prolapses) when it closes. That makes some blood flow backward from the ventricle to the atrium and causes a heart murmur. It's seldom serious, but it requires an antibiotic prior to each dental visit to prevent infection that could damage the valve.

The antibiotic for MVP reduces but doesn't eliminate the tenderness inside my cheek. It also lessens the inflammation and allows the dentist to dismiss the lesion as a benign *Lichen Planus* that does not require further investigation.

But I grow anxious because this problem has become chronic. I go to a dermatologist for a second opinion. He agrees with the dentist's diagnosis of *Lichen Planus*. Still worried and dissatisfied with this easy dismissal, I decide to seek one more opinion. My anxiety level is unbearable.

As a student, Marie had worked in my office and now has her own dermatology practice. She is loved and respected by all, and for good reason. One look in my mouth and she promptly marches me down the hall, hand in hand, to a dental surgeon affectionately referred to as Uncle Jim. He immediately schedules me for a biopsy the next day, a Friday, after my office hours. I can't remember a day in the office fraught with more anxiety.

Jim operates under local anesthesia, injecting painful needles in my mouth and neck. His nurse assistant pries open my mouth with metal pliers and stretches my mouth until it feels like it will become unhinged. I imagine I will never be able to close it again. The procedure seems to take an unusually long time, and the amount of my cheek that Jim removes is unexpected The specimen is the size of a small nectarine. I can't tell how much of my cheek is left because of the packing to stem the bleeding, but I feel that only a layer of skin must remain.

In a few days I return for Uncle Jim to check the surgical site and give me a diagnosis. I meet a distressed Uncle Jim, leaning against the wall for support.

"Gert, I was so sure it was benign that I almost didn't send the tissue to the lab." The diagnosis is so unexpected that I am stunned, speechless. Squamous cell carcinoma, the type of cancer found in smokers, drinkers, and people with poor dental care, for none of which am I guilty.

Uncle Jim is very kind. He embraces me and allows me a few moments to cry and compose myself. We decide that I should see the oncologic surgeon who performs cancer surgery for my patients.

Monday, Christmas Eve 1997, fortunately gives me a light day in the office. That evening I meet with the oncologic surgeon and a plastic surgeon. After studying the slide in the pathology laboratory, they have decided that, since the lesion is only seven-tenths of a centimeter, they can simply do a local excision and I can be discharged in two days. The only required study is the negative chest x-ray that I obtain that afternoon.

Not as awful as I had expected. Since it's Christmas Eve, I do not call Marie, my dermatologist to report until Wednesday morning, the day after Christmas. Her response is immediate and upsetting.

"What? No MRI? No blood work? That is entirely unsatisfactory."

"Marie, you have to help me now. I don't know whom to see. This is such an unusual lesion and unusual site. Can you suggest someone who has had some experience with this and whom you trust?"

She gives me three names. I rule out the first because, in trying to get help for his mother who was my patient, both he and his wife refused to respond. I had called them several times when the mother was calling neighbors, also my patients, at 3 A.M. almost nightly. He was finally forced to step in when his mother set her apartment on fire.

The second doctor had been ungracious and unresponsive to patients, including my brother, who I had previously referred to him. I choose the third name, a doctor who is very highly recommended but unknown to me. Dr. H. is a skilled surgeon, imported from Canada five years earlier to set up the first head and neck cancer department at the University of Pennsylvania. Because of hospital politics, he very recently moved to a different institution. I can't find him in the phone book and immediately panic. Has he left the city?

I finally locate him at his new office. With my diagnosis, I am given an immediate appointment. My daughter Joan comes with me to his office where we are greeted warmly and sympathetically. He takes lots of time to discuss the lesion with us but says, "I will not examine you or proceed without your first obtaining an MRI, a gastroscopy, and a bronchoscopy that I will perform myself. This lesion not infrequently will appear simultaneously in the lung and the stomach."

That was a startling revelation. Much worse than Marie or I imagined.

"I won't take a chance of operating in your mouth without first checking these two organs."

What a potential disaster if I'd chosen the first surgeon! I've never heard of a surgeon, a specialist in cancer surgery of the head and neck, doing his own invasive studies of the GI and pulmonary organs. I feel reassured by his thoroughness, but the prospect of an MRI is almost as daunting as the cancer diagnosis because I am severely claustrophobic. I can't even sit in the middle or window seat of an airplane.

Joan is allowed into the room that houses a gigantic, roaring, throbbing MRI machine. She massages my legs and talks to me before the deafening machine noise begins.

"Mom, imagine you are at the top of the ski slope. The sun is shining. Packed powder, no moguls, no snowboarders, no other skiers on the hill."

"Joanie, I am so upset I can only think of being at the top of a double Black Diamond and scared shitless. Please talk about something else."

She rubs my legs very hard, causing some pain that helps divert my attention, until I inadvertently open my eyes in the middle of the procedure. The MRI casement looks less than three inches above my nose. Through a small window, I can see the technician sitting high up above the machine, watching me. I almost stop the procedure. By keeping my eyes scrunched closed, I am able to get through the exam. The noise is ear splitting. (In these earlier days of MRIs, ear protectors or soothing music aren't routinely supplied.) Joanie's reassurance during the off periods helps my control.

When the gurney slides out of the machine, it is drenched in my sweat. It's the longest hour I can recall and one I won't soon forget. I vow to be even more careful before ordering an MRI for my patients. For the many subsequent procedures, I will come saturated with tranquilizers.

The next steps, a bronchoscopy and gastroscopy, are performed under anaesthesia and personally by Dr. H. As I wait in the recovery room for the verdict, he walks in still gowned. He swipes off his cap, waves it in the air, and smiles.

"The tests were negative, and I will call Joan to let her know."

"I do have a daughter in Philadelphia, too, so you don't have to call Joan in Massachusetts."

"Joan was the daughter who came to the office with you and therefore I will call her."

I am so touched by his sensitivity in the midst of my fear and anxiety. I feel lucky to have put my life in his hands.

The surgical date was quickly set. The perfunctory preoperative examination to rule out any change or any acute infection takes just a few minutes. It is performed by the top honcho, his chief Fellow, who says, "You may wake up with a tube in your neck."

I dismiss this comment as unlikely because all the pre-op studies have been negative for metastases. But after thirteen and a half hours on the operating table, I indeed return to intensive care with a tracheotomy tube hanging out of my neck.

Both daughters—frightened, haggard, tired, and anxious— await me. Having been unconscious for so many hours, I am not tired but I am upset by their appearance. I can't talk to reassure them so I motion for a clipboard and pencil. I cannot bend my face and swollen neck to see to write. They hold the board up in front of my nose. I only have one functioning arm and, with blurry eyes, I manage to print some funny limericks to assure them that I am okay and still have a sense of humor. Despite what must be my frightening appearance, I try to make them smile.

> "There once was a mother from Bala
> Who fled from the halls of Valhalla
> With the aid of her kids
> Who supplied her with skids
> She slid out with a whoop and a holla."

They smile. I later learn that Dr. H. had told Barbie, when I first arrived from the OR, "Take that look off your face or you'll scare your mother to death."

Joanie had worked in a hospital OR so she is not as visibly shocked. I regain feeling over the next few hours but remain sleepless

and restless after thirteen hours asleep under anaesthesia. I'm
especially anxious. I am sure I will die by choking on my own
saliva, so I ring my buzzer for frequent aspirations of the tracheal
tube. My sympathetic, attentive, and considerate nurse cautions
her relief, a very young man, by whispering, "Don't let her make
you aspirate her too often because it will irritate her trachea."

Overhearing this, I am sure I will drown in my own secretions.
I will choke, unable to breathe, the mucus obstructing the tracheal
tube, and now a relief nurse is being warned to respond less
frequently to my calls for help!

To allay my anxiety, Dr. H. has told my daughters that I could
survive for many hours with a "blocked tube." But I am not
reassured. For the first twenty-four hours, I remain in what is intensive-
intensive care. Then I move to another section of the floor to simple
intensive care where I stay for sixteen days instead of being transferred
to the surgical floor. Dr. H. feels that the nurses in this section, whom
he has personally trained, are more capable and able to respond more
knowledgeably to prevent any complications.

This section is so noisy with emergency bells sounding over
twenty-four hours. I get little sleep, especially because I have to
remain sitting up at all times. I'm constantly anxious that I'll slump
down while asleep and pull out all the tubes connecting me to the
life-sustaining hardware.

The operative procedure has removed a large portion of what
was left of the inner portion of my right cheek. To fill the hole,
tendons, muscle, and blood vessels from my left forearm are used
to fill out the cheek. A thin skin graft from my right thigh is taken
and placed over the operative site on my forearm to aid in healing.
Dr. H. has taken the precaution preoperatively to learn that I need
my right arm to play tennis if, in fact, I will ever be able to return
to such activity. He also puts a flap of skin on the right side of my
neck where he'd removed the cancerous cervical glands to serve as
a signal if the graft starts being rejected in my mouth. This area
could more readily be checked by the nurses rather than going

into the mouth as needed every two hours. If the signal graft does not take on the neck, Dr. H. has only two hours to get me back up on the operating table to try to save the inner cheek graft.

I have surprisingly little pain. The only discomfort is not being able to lie down.I am fed through a gastric tube that is threaded through my right nostril and passed into my stomach. Unfortunately the nutritionist calculates the feeding for a man weighing 170 pounds. I gain an amazing six pounds on gastric feeding. She later apologizes, but it's too late for the weight gain.

Intravenous treatment is placed in the blood vessel of my right arm. The left arm is immobilized in an open cast to aid healing. For a while I am unable to scratch an itch. Every morning three doctors work on me simultaneously: One in my mouth and neck, another on my arm, and the third on my thigh from which the skin graft had been removed. I feel like the Soutine dog, eviscerated, all limbs extended, drawn and quartered.

My daughters greet my visitors in the hallway and forewarn them so that they will not be appalled at my grotesque appearance and frighten me with their reactions. I have not yet seen a mirror. Several of my visitors look so pale and upset when they approach my bed. I assume it is because of the networks of tubes and bottles encasing me. I can only reassure them by whispers after occluding the trach opening.

Several days later, when I am finally able to walk, I look in the mirror on the wall and become scared and terrified. From my right eye down to the clavicle the swollen distortion is horrific. I look disfigured, like a lopsided elephant man. I am reluctant to walk out of the room because I'm fearful of frightening other patients on the floor.

Despite the MRI's being negative, Dr. H has discovered cancerous microscopic infiltration of the maxilla, two submandibular glands, a border of my tongue, and three cervical glands. He removes part of the maxilla, several teeth, and part of my tongue as well. How lucky I am to be in his hands.

My chief concern during this weird period in the hospital is choking on my own secretions. The only medication I need after this very extensive surgery is a sleeping pill to try to get some sleep while sitting up to relieve my fear of choking to death. The only pain I suffer is when the doctor removes the gastric feeding tube. The tube has been in place for two weeks and adhesions have formed along its track. They are torn as the tube is extracted. A weird and painful experience, it feels like the lining of my nose and esophagus are being pulled out along with the tube.

Yet the removal of the trach tube is an unbelievable relief. I can finally talk. For many days after surgery I could not talk at all. I would cover the breathing tube and whisper. I'd tap two times for *yes*, once for *no*. The funniest call is the first, from a nephew in Grenoble, France.

"Here I am in the bathroom, in my jockey shorts, in the middle of the night, looking out at the snow-covered mountains, talking to myself on the telephone with someone across the ocean tapping on the receiver."

I am finally discharged, but I still need to sleep sitting up. Joan, meanwhile, has been taught how to aspirate me should an emergency arise at home. A large aspirator has been delivered to my house before my arrival. This huge machine sits threateningly at my bedside. A frightening but potentially life saving piece of equipment.

We cannot relax this first night at home. I'm certainly unable to sleep, though thoroughly exhausted. Finally Joanie climbs into bed with me and we both take a sleeping pill—to no avail. After several hours, we both take a Benadryl that produces a feeling of euphoria and unsteadiness to the point of making us stagger and hold on to the walls to get to the bathroom. Finally we pass out into a drug-induced stupor.

Having survived the first night, we know we can make it. We fortunately never use the aspirator. We manage to get me into the bathtub, in three inches of water, without getting any essential areas wet. My arms and legs are propped up and hang over the side of the tub. My first bath in three weeks is so much better than a bed wash. A nurse comes every morning for weeks to cleanse and dress the involved areas.

I cannot chew or even swallow very well. I only take very soft watery foods, bland liquids, and no pills for six weeks. I survive on creamed spinach and mushy oatmeal. It takes two weeks at home and a physician friend to convince Barbie that I should be allowed to walk down the flight of stairs alone. I could not have survived without the care of my devoted daughters.

After two weeks at home, I face the first post-op visit to the surgeon and I'm numb with fear.

"The good news is that the margins of the lesion in the cheek and mouth are clear, but the maxilla and glands were positive," he begins. "As I told you, Gert, I rarely see a case where there has not already been metastatic spread. These were only microscopic infiltrations and therefore were not picked up by the MRI, but I took the nodes and the lab reported them positive."

How lucky to have picked an experienced surgeon. How unlucky that I have metastases.

Seven weeks of daily radiation treatment follow under a deafening dinosaur monster machine. A rigid perforated plastic mask is fashioned to fit over my face, head, and neck. The mask is then screwed down with clamps so that my head cannot move. My tongue has to fit sideways into a slot in the mask so that the radiation can hit the operative site.

My poor prognosis, the surgery, its aftermath, the many weeks of daily radiation therapy, the worry that I may not be able to carry on, the anxiety, the responsibility of providing continuing care to my patients . . . all result in the worst decision of my medical life.

I sell my practice, not to an HMO but to a major hospital system.

* * *

I am writing this seven years after the surgery. I am still checked regularly, but all is, fortunately, negative to date.

13

Patient Perils

My face and neck are grotesquely deformed after major surgery for cancer. With a poor prognosis, I do not know when or if I ever will be able to return full time to my office.

In 1999, I make one of the greatest mistakes of my life.

I've practiced medicine for forty-eight years. I've taken care of three generations in several families among my thousands of patients. I am anxious to ensure their continuity of care. I therefore sell my practice not a "managed care" organization but to a local hospital health system. A colleague will be assigned to join me in the office and will be prepared to take over if illness forces me to leave. Fortunately the choice of a colleague is mine.

I have just met a wonderful physician who was recently discharged from a failing HMO facility. Lez is a great doctor, a great athlete, and a lucky find. She has a terrific sense of humor. We work and play wonderfully well together. I recover faster than expected and return to the office. I'm still swollen but not so grotesque that my appearance frightens patients. I explain that I had a badly infected wisdom tooth with involvement of my neck and jaw.

After two and a half weeks of post-op recovery, the trach tube is finally removed. Then another six weeks of daily radiation and I've made a miraculous comeback. I sign a contract for one year with the hospital health system. The ensuing year is wonderful, although my salary is low in contrast to other physicians in the system. My attorney has not been forceful and I, still recuperating, accept the inadequate terms because I'm so happy to resume work for however long I can last. Alice, the purchasing agency's business representative, later remarks on the meager pay: "We've never paid a doctor so little."

Practicing medicine now, however, is happily free of the burden of paperwork that the agency now takes over. For years I had spent hours every evening filling out forms, coding diagnoses by numbers instead of words, which was double the work and totally nonproductive busywork to meet the demands of government bureaucracy.

I have no HMO patients in my practice. My patients pay for their health insurance privately. They do not leave me to join the highly seductive, deceptive HMO systems. Many patients are well aware of the shortcomings of HMOs and often report receiving as many as five telephone calls in one day from five different HMO's trying to convince them to join with all sorts of attractive offers, including a meal at an expensive restaurant. And no wonder, the government pays the HMO's $5,000 yearly for each Medicare enrollee, whether or not seen in the office. This payment varies from state to state.

My experience with the managed care system comes from contacts with my colleagues. In starting a new practice, Lez has many patients from the HMO system. For each one, she must refer to catalogs to see which tests and procedures are allowed. Every HMO has its own regulations. Some change the rules without notifying physicians in time to cancel the now-disallowed tests. Without such proper notification, patients are billed for tests that had been previously covered. Fortunately, these are not my problems.

Lez and I enjoy a wonderful partnership. I feel well at the end of my one-year contract and sign a renewal for another year. But this second year is a disaster for the hospital corporation. Reimbursement is reduced across the board—from Medicare, HMOs, and all the insurance companies.

Health care corporations, top-heavy with administrators and inadequate ancillary personnel, become less profitable. Although my agency is not an HMO, it accepts enrolled patients. It also suffers decreased revenue and therefore closes several offices— including mine after the end of my contract. Several physicians from a few of the offices are transferred to a single suite at the local hospital. My patients' records are to be sent there and stored for patients to retrieve later. With each physician having his or her own medical assistant and telephone-answering secretary, chaos ensues.

The combined office is run like a factory but much less efficiently. Requested charts, misfiled by poorly trained, undereducated and underpaid ancillary personnel, cannot be found. Machines answer the telephone, rarely a human voice. After a long wait, callers may be told, "If you want to make a call, hang up and call again." Calls that do get through to the voicemail are often not returned for hours, days, or frequently not all. Several patients threaten legal action to get their charts. One patient does engage an attorney. This kind of inadequate service is reported repeatedly in managed care and corporate facilities.

Patients call me for help. It is difficult for them to find a suitable physician, and particularly difficult to find an obstetrician/gynecologist. Many are leaving the area or medicine itself because of impossibly high malpractice insurance premiums. Outrageously high premiums drive 900 physicians from Pennsylvania in one year.

One patient, given the names of three gynecologists, discovers that one is entering a psychiatry residency, another has apparently just quit and left her office without a forwarding address, and the third will not take a new patient for four months. Gynecologists are only performing office procedures, no surgery, because of insurance rates. Obstetricians are quitting practice because their insurance rates as high as a surgeon's, despite obstetricians' much lower yearly income.

Physicians in many other specialties leave the state, retire at an earlier age, or go into other fields because of these dramatic negative

changes, particularly the exorbitant cost of malpractice insurance.
Other contributing factors are the mountains of unnecessary
paperwork, restrictions shortening office time to fifteen minutes
and one-symptom visits (that is, don't come in with both chest
pains *and* a broken leg on the same visit), limits on testing and
referrals, restrictions on hospital admissions and length of hospital
stay, denied laboratory tests, and x-rays to be done only at company
facilities, which frequently cause dangerous delays for the patient.

The result? Poor patient care is added to the unbelievable,
ever-present specter of crippling malpractice suits. A Philadelphia
jury in 1999 awards one plaintiff $10 million in a malpractice
suit. In that year alone, more money is awarded in malpractice
litigation in Philadelphia in only six months than in the entire
state of California in one year.

My office colleague Lez, a wonderful, empathetic, and brilliant
physician, has two malpractice suits pending. Both are trivial and
basically do not involve her. She has not seen the suing patient for
five years. She has to meet with attorneys and travel out of state.
This not only a waste of time, but it is always anxiety-producing.
Both cases are eventually thrown out-of-court. Plaintiffs' attorneys
sue everyone within reach so that the malpractice insurance of as
many physicians as possible can be charged to reach the maximum
assignment.

The atmosphere is such that it is difficult to attract physicians
to this city. Not only are scores of doctors leaving the area, but
many jobs also cannot be filled. Positions, such as those in trauma
units and emergency rooms, are high risk so some physicians in
those areas cannot get insurance and others get it only with
impossibly high premiums. Many Philadelphia trauma units close
and particularly high-risk surgical physicians flee. One hospital in
Delaware loses its entire staff of orthopedic surgeons.

Patients are dropped from HMO rolls because they need
expensive treatment. HMOs abandon Medicare patients, leaving
them without coverage, because government reimbursement is too
low for HMOs to make their huge profits. Some 150,000 Medicare
patients, dropped in New Jersey in 2002, are stranded without

insurance. Women with breast cancer have to sue for treatment. Women are being discharged within twenty-four hours after radical breast surgery because their insurance will not cover a longer hospital stay, even though it's medically necessary. New mothers are sent home the day of delivery until increasing reports of newborn distress and deaths force a change in that dangerous policy.

My friend Mike has a patient with colon cancer. Al needs highly toxic medications postoperatively that should only be administered by a specially trained oncologist. But in Al's case, an untrained primary physician gives the medicines because a primary doctor is less expensive. Still working to support his family, Al has to travel several towns away to receive appropriate radiation therapy because no other radiation facility contracted with his HMO is closer to his hometown. Al later needs chest surgery, but the HMO refuses to cover the procedure at his well-trained surgeon's hospital because the HMO has no contract with that hospital—meaning it gets no kickback. The HMO only allows the surgery at its inadequately equipped, small community hospital that is inexperienced with the potentially life-saving operation that could prolong Al's life.

His surgery is performed, when Al pays for it himself. He later files suit against the HMO for reimbursement. Having a friend on the Board of Directors of this insurance company helps Al win his suit. Would that we all could be this lucky.

I meet Tommy in the waiting room when we are both going through our first weeks of radiation for cancer. An eighteen-year-old with a brain cancer, Tommy had an MRI ordered by his radiation oncologist to determine whether and at what site this advancing lesion will require radiation therapy. The record of his MRI, performed at his HMO facility, was lost. A second MRI was performed at the same facility. Again the records are lost, resulting in a three-week delay of treatment that can affect his chances for survival.

Susan, the office nurse whom I've gotten to know well after two months of my own daily radiation, tells me almost tearfully, "I pleaded with the insurer to allow Tommy to be sent to another facility because of the urgency. They refused again. They'd only allow him to return for a third time to their facility. And they pay that facility each time even though the records get lost!"

Despite the lost records and delays, Tommy does well and lives another two years.

My patient, Betty, is tested for Lyme disease two days before she moves to California. When her results come in positive, she has already departed without leaving a forwarding address. After forty-eight hours of calling her friends in Philadelphia, I finally locate her in Long Beach, California. I call the local pharmacy there to order her medication.

The pharmacist asks me, "Can I pick your brains? My brother, a well-known photojournalist in Nebraska, was dropped by his HMO because his treatment got too expensive. He developed Lyme disease with neurologic involvement that now requires intravenous therapy for several weeks. We don't know what to do since he doesn't have coverage."

"He should be in a hospital," I tell her. "I would advise you to get him in as soon as possible."

Several months later she calls to ask me to be an expert witness in their suit against the HMO. "I would be happy to come," I explain. "But the courts require the expert witness to be a specialist. The testimony of a general practitioner like me would not be acceptable." With the appropriate treatment, I learn later, he does recover.

Beatrice, a young woman whom I treated through high school and college, is now employed by an insurance company with its own HMO coverage. Over a period of six days, Beatrice calls her HMO doctor's office three times with complaints of increasing pelvic pain and leaves messages, but there's no response to her calls. Her mother, who is also my patient, persuades Beatrice to see me even though I am not in her HMO's system or "network."

Nothing is worse—potentially as a surgical emergency—than severe pelvic pain and tenderness in a young woman, particularly at 5:30 P.M. on a summer Friday. I call her HMO, but no one is available on her panel of participating doctors.

Luckily one of my own patients is a gynecologist in Beatrice's HMO system. When I reach her, she is still in her office and agrees to see Beatrice right away. Beatrice overhears our phone conversation. When I hang up, I find her in tears. "You're going to be okay, Beatrice. You'll be able to become pregnant even if you require surgery. The surgery, if necessary, will be safe and curative."

"That's not why I'm crying. Suppose I had not come back to you?" she says between sobs.

Since retiring after fifty years of practice, I find conditions have become progressively worse. Finding and trying to make an appointment with a physician whom one fondly refers to as "an old-time physician" is well nigh impossible in today's healthcare system. Almost all are working under the constraints of limited time for office visits and referrals only to often inadequate facilities of the profit-motivated employing agency. Those physicians who do not conform do not have their contracts renewed. Many doctors are working to improve the medical system, but only 600,000 physicians are practicing in the United States today (2003). This situation therefore requires all of the over 200 million people in our country to bring back a more people-friendly responsible system of delivering medical care.

14

Herman

As a healthy young adolescent, Herman was incarcerated in Auschwitz. He survived for three years. He had no formal education beyond his fourteenth year. When he was liberated at age seventeen, Herman was unskilled, unprepared to support himself, and without any living relatives. He was one of the fortunate people, however, because he was healthy enough to enter a rehabilitation program, the Organization for Rehabilitation and Training.

ORT was a Jewish settlement established in Cyprus as a displaced persons camp to help train concentration camp survivors. There he met Genia who became his wife. Both were orphans, having lost their entire Munich families in the camps. Herman became a skilled woodworker in Cyprus. Later, with the help of international agencies, both he and Genia arrived in Philadelphia where he was able to start a new life as a cabinet maker.

Herman, Genia, and their two sons become my patients. When my family moves to a new house in 1967, I employ Herman to construct our built-in shelves and cabinets. While he hammers and stains, we talk for many hours about his past life, his childhood in Munich, his experiences in Cyprus. But he never speaks of his years in Auschwitz, nor do I ask him. I feel this was a period too painful for him to dredge up.

But I keep haranguing him about the Vietnam War. This is the late 1960s. I try to convince Herman to participate in the anti-war protests, particularly since his two sons might shortly be drafted.

"You must be aware of the terrible atrocities? The horrors being reported? The many Americans being killed? We're burning villages, destroying their farms, planting mines, and killing farmers, women, and children. Aren't you aware of the public protests trying to end this?" I badger him.

This goes on for hours, whenever I'm home and he is working quietly. Finally he stops his staining and turns toward me with irritation and anger in his voice:

"Please stop! It doesn't concern me. You can't reach me!"

"But it concerns all of us," I persist. "Soon your sons may be drafted to take part in these terrible crimes. We are all responsible."

"Dr. C . . ." Then, silent for a moment, he sighs deeply, hesitantly. "Do you think your horror stories can affect me? Do you know how I survived Auschwitz? I worked for the Nazis. I was fourteen, strong, young, healthy. How I survived? I worked for the murderers every day for three years. I pulled dead bodies out of the crematoria and piled them two stories, sometimes three stories, high. You're telling *me* horror stories?"

Herman's eyes glisten with unshed tears. I also become tearful and silent, guilty at having caused such distress.

"I'm sorry, so sorry, Herman. Forgive me." I can say no more. I am appalled at my insensitivity.

We silently share a cup of coffee and I leave him with his sandpaper and stains.

15

Ruth

My favorite biking path winds along the Schuylkill River. I've ridden this path since I was twelve years old, but the scenery on the west bank has taken on a different significance in recent decades. Whenever boxcars pass on the adjacent railroad track, I sadly recall the transports of Jews to concentration camps in cars like these. Some of the surivors are my present patients. To this day, this horrible image is conjured up.

I try to ride several days a week. This is the closest and safest path, which allows me to ride on an occasional midday hour or after office hours when daylight is longer. I most often ride after hours on Fridays because they tend to be shorter workdays.

On this Friday afternoon, I have just ended a distressing visit with a new patient in room two. Jane has a cancer diagnosis that is unsuspected in so young a woman. She and I are understandably upset. The last patient waits in room three. With a feeling of relief, I knock and enter to examine Ruth. I expect to see her well coiffed, fashionably dressed, and upbeat with her usual slightly askew smile. I am greeted instead by a sad, disheveled, distressed woman. Her face is drawn, her head bowed, her eyes brimming with unshed tears. Even when ill with infection, fever, coughing with chest pain, or generally feeling lousy, Ruth never appears in such a state as this.

My first thought is of her family. Is someone seriously ill or was there some terrible accident? Ruth would not respond to her own personal problems with such distress.

"Is something wrong with your husband or your children, Ruth?"

"No, it's nothing like that," she answers in muffled tones.

"Are you in pain?" I encircle her shoulder and feel her forehead with my free hand. It's not hot.

She remains silent. Finally after taking a deep breath, she manages to say, "I can't do it. I am so upset." A deep sigh. "But I can't refuse to do it."

I take her hands in mine, "Take your time. I have plenty of time. You are my last patient today." I place a box of Kleenex next to her. "Is it someone in your family? Does someone need your help?"

"Oh, no, nothing like that. I would never refuse anyone in my family."

"So what can be so terrible?" I make somewhat idle comments to try to get her to relax so that she can talk to me. Finally, her voice gets calmer and stronger.

"I am being asked to tell how I survived during the Holocaust."

"Why the distress now? I don't understand why this upsets you so much," I ask. "You and I have talked about the Holocaust without so much discomfiture."

"This is different. Tonight at Oneg Shabbat, at my synagogue, members who are survivors of the Holocaust are being asked to tell their stories of how they survived. I can't do it. My two granddaughters will be in the audience and I cannot tell them of my terror, of being hidden three years in a locked closet in an attic. I've never told them the whole story."

I am shocked at this revelation. Ruth has never told me the whole story either, although we've talked many times of that period. When she is finally able to talk more calmly, she takes deep breaths and wipes her eyes with the offered sheets of Kleenex.

"I will tell you why I can't tell them, and see what you think. I had a best friend at school, Anna, a Polish girl, not Jewish. We were in the same class for five years. Our families were good friends, celebrating holidays and vacations together until I was twelve years old and my world was destroyed. Anna's family lived just outside what was to become the walled-in 'Warsaw ghetto.' We were all aware of the impending doom, but my family did not have the means to escape. We knew that shortly we would not be allowed to walk out through the walled enclosures soon to surround the ghetto."

Ruth stops and gasps. Tears spill down her cheeks. I hold her hand as she tries to continue. I wipe her tears, barely holding back my own. We have spent long hours talking about her childhood in Poland, but she has never told me these details. Her high blood pressure and gastric problems are related to her past, as we both recognize, but she has never revealed to me these very terrible personal experiences.

I tell Pauline, my secretary, to hold all my calls. We are not to be interrupted. I sit silently and give Ruth time to collect herself.

"My mother realized that any moment now the ghetto would be totally fenced in, and no one would be able to leave without inspection and permission by the guards. She bagged everything of value she could carry—rings, a silver candelabra handed down from her grandmother, valuable jewelry—and we carried them to Clara, Anna's mother. My mother begged Clara as a mother, as a friend, to take me and hide me until it was safe for a Jew to walk again in the streets of Poland. Our two mothers held each other crying. They knew this would be the last time they would see each other. Clara took me in.

"I survived by hiding in a locked closet in the attic of their house for three years. Anna and the rest of her family were unaware of my hiding place. My presence was a danger to the entire family, but Clara took this chance to save me. She allowed me out of the closet in the middle of the night, when everyone was asleep, to stretch. She brought me food and water to wash inside the closet. I had to move my bowels in a paper bag, which she carried out and buried in the field. So closely was everyone watched that I never in three years used a toilet. I never left the attic.

"My granddaughters have never been told this story. They will be in the audience this evening. I cannot tell them how I suffered. I feel so torn and guilty, but I feel I owe it to those who saved me and to those who did not survive. I owe it to the brave Poles, few as they were, to tell of the heroism of this one woman, Clara."

Silent, mournful, and exhausted after this painful revelation, we continue to hold hands and look into each other's eyes, speechless. After more tissues and a hug, we are both finally calmer.

"Ruth, I understand your reluctance to tell your granddaughters of your suffering. I agree with you that it would cause them great pain. Perhaps you would feel more comfortable omitting some of the personal, most painful details and, instead, telling them about the woman who saved you, the threat to her family, her daughter, and what would have happened to them were you discovered," I suggest.

After a long thoughtful pause, her little crooked smile lights up her face and her tears dry. "I think I can handle that. I can talk about Clara, how she scrounged food from herself and her family to feed me, how she stayed up all hours of the night to comfort me, how she mended her daughters cast-off clothes to keep me warm."

We embrace and Ruth leaves after a cursory examination. Snow has started to fall and it is late. I sit for a while and think of my many patients, refugees who also took years to be able to describe their horrors. I feel warmed by my wonderfully cluttered walls hung with thank-you gifts from my patients. Many are from Genia, an Auschwitz graduate: Her framed, colorful needlepoint gifts, always containing *Shalom* woven into each picture. She was incarcerated as an adolescent. Today she still cannot drive through New Jersey because farm silos remind her of the Auschwitz crematoria where her entire family burned. She and her family were transported to Auschwitz in just such windowless, airless boxcars that line the tracks on West River Drive.

Now as I cycle along the drive, I observe with pleasure the dozens of Japanese cherry blossom trees changing in color and size daily. The brilliant forsythia spread wildly, luxuriantly, along the banks of the river. The newly planted magnolia trees form purple cups. The first harbingers of spring lighten but do not erase the memories.

16

Genia

Genia waits in office #3. She is a forceful, buxom, ruddy-faced, middle-aged, middle-class, religious mother of two teenagers. A two-pack-a-day smoker. Someone I have not been able to help.

"Now I can't even walk one level block from 53rd to 54th Street without having to stop because of terrible cramps in my legs."

"Genia, I am sorry, but I've told you before that I can't help your pain if you don't stop smoking. Try the system we have talked about. I am sure it can work for you."

"Can't you give me a pill to help me? It's hard for me to believe that you can't just give me a pill. I can't stop smoking. It's the only thing that helps my nerves," she pleads.

"There is no pill to stop smoking, Genia, Of course, I can give you a pill for your nerves, but that won't stop your smoking. Try my plan to stop, and you'll be amazed at how quickly the leg cramps decrease."

"*Ich ken nicht.* I can't. I'm addicted. It's like schnapps."

I can sympathize with Genia. I recognize her difficulty, but trying to help her is so difficult. Quitting smoking is not a question of will.

A childhood memory flashes: I recall a man on a flat board, supported on wheels at its four corners. His legs are amputated, his body missing below his buttocks. Dirty heavy pads encase his hands that he uses to propel his board along the pavement. He is stationed regularly in front of Claflin's Shoe Store, 16th and Chestnut Streets, where he begs. I pass him every Saturday morning on my way to piano lessons at the Presser Building. I am ten-years-old, so grown up, busing into town myself.

Worrying about Genia and perseverating, as I so often do when the problem seems without solution, remind me of this man and how impossible it was for him to stop smoking.

I meet him years later when I am a medical resident at St. Luke's Hospital where he's been admitted for removal of one arm. Smoking has so seriously impaired the blood supply to his arm that it must be amputated.

"Would you believe it?" an amazed orderly reports, "that poor sucker tried to bribe me to go out and buy him cigarettes!"

Smoking is truly addictive, as powerful as any street drug. I appreciate Genia's struggle even more when I recall this sad, crippled man.

Genia still carries the accent of her birthplace, Germany, and frequently lapses into Yiddish, her native tongue. Her early childhood was spent in a large, religious, closely knit Jewish family in Munich where a woman smoking was *verboten,* I'm sure. Genia spent her adolescence in Auschwitz but lost her entire family. As a sole survivor, she was never able to talk to me or probably to anyone about these years in the camp except to say, "I can't drive through New Jersey without having nightmares. The silos look like the crematoria of the camp."

Genia returns to my office four months later. "I really didn't believe you, but it's true. First I cut down, then I was finally able to stop smoking altogether after a couple months. I had to quit because I couldn't stop coughing, and finally I couldn't catch my breath even when I didn't walk. The cough was unbearable. My chest hurt just to breath, and my family complained constantly of my smell. I can now walk more than one block, and it's getting better all the time."

"So how did you do it?" I ask her.

"When I felt I couldn't control myself, I went outside as you suggested. But I couldn't smoke out of doors because I was ashamed—it was a *shanda*. I couldn't let my neighbors see me smoking." (This occurs in the 1960s when the sight of a woman smoking in public, especially a middle-aged Jewish woman, is not widely acceptable.)

Breaking into a smile, Genia says, "But now what do I do about getting fat?"

"I'm so proud of you," I say as we embrace. "That problem we can easily handle together."

Genia's husband and two sons are delighted at her victory over smoking, and their house also smells so much better.

17

Archie # 1: Securinega Suffruticosa

Archie's story, told in the following three installments, chronicles the experimental use of a little-known Chinese herbal medicine that extended and improved the life of a brave University of Pennsylvania professor who suffered from a disease for which there is no known treatment or cure to date.

"Mom, did you hear NPR this morning?"

"You just woke me up. What happened?"

"An amazing government announcement! Thousands of Gulf War veterans from the first Bush's war are showing up with ALS. Isn't that what Archie had?"

"Yes. What? Are you sure they said thousands?"

"Yes, the news was released from the NIH and was well documented."

"Wow! Did they say anything about treatment? Are you sure it was ALS? Did they describe it?" I am now fully awake.

"No, just the bald announcement."

"Thanks for calling. I'll check it out."

Shocked by the announcement, I jump out of bed.

Amyotrophic Lateral Sclerosis (ALS), commonly known as Lou Gehrig's disease, is a previously rare disease of unknown etiology. That was its status in 1969 when my friend Archie, a sociology professor at University of Pennsylvania, was diagnosed with the disease. At that time, fewer than 4,000 people with ALS were alive in the United States in any given year. As with all ALS patients Archie's life expectancy was estimated to be three to five years from the time of diagnosis. There was no known treatment. News that the disease is now appearing in the thousands is shocking. In my fifty years of practice, Archie is the only person whom I know with ALS.

We meet at a dinner party in the 1968 soon after he arrives at the University. He is handsome, tanned, and muscular, with the body of a well-trained athlete. We discover that we've both just read Theodore Roszak's new book *The Making of a Counter Culture*, and we concur that it's the best exposition of 1960s in print. To the exclusion of the other guests, we spend most of the evening discussing those tumultuous times. I find him charming, without affectation, very bright and politically aware—just the kind of man to whom I am immediately attracted.

The turmoil of the 1960s remains a source of constant anxiety on a national and personal level, and Archie and I share similar worries. We and our children are very much involved in anti-Vietnam war protests. Before each march, other physicians and I are instructed in the treatment of tear gas attacks and police brutality, which heightens our worry for the safety of our kids. Both our families have been in all sorts of picket lines, school discrimination protests, and peace marches, many marked by police violence.

"I didn't expect such liberal attitudes from a physician" is Archie's parting comment as we say goodbye that night. I know that we both feel an immediate kinship.

We do not meet again for several months. In the interim, Felice, a mutual friend and Archie's colleague, informs me that about two months after his arrival at the university, he appears to be ill. He has lost a considerable amount of weight and developed a slow, shuffling gait. He has fallen several times, fractured his wrist, and often comes to class with bruises. Archie has spoken to no one about these changes, and people are reluctant to probe or offer help for fear of offending him.

In 1970, eighteen months after our first meeting, Archie calls me. I do not recognize his voice, which is noticeably weak and hesitant.

"Can you meet me in my office for lunch?" he asks. Three days later when I walk into his office my face must reflect my horror at his appearance. This cannot be the handsome vigorous man I had met less than two years ago. How could these drastic changes have taken place in such a short time? His pale skin is taut, bloodless, almost transparent, and he looks skeletal. His right arm hangs limply, lifeless, at his side. Both hands are swollen to twice their normal size, which only accentuates his thin, wasted appearance. His coat is slung over his shoulders like a cape. I guess that he is unable to reach his arms into the sleeves. I cannot imagine what has caused such striking changes other than an advancing terminal disease. He has to have noticed my reaction but makes no comment, and I am not comfortable asking. What a contrast to the candor we enjoyed at our first meeting.

We set out for the Faculty Club for lunch. Hardly lifting his feet, he shuffles along the uneven pavement. I am fearful he'll fall, but I cannot offer help to this proud, reticent professor. He must recognize my mounting distress, which I am barely able to contain, but he makes no comment. During the meal, I notice that Archie can hold food on his fork, but has to use both hands to grasp his glass and lift it unsteadily to his mouth. Lunch is surreal as we both try to sustain a normal conversation.

After the unrelieved ordeal of the meal, he finally says with remarkable composure, "I feel from our previous meeting that I could ask you to help me." A long silence follows as he takes a deep breath. His voice is barely audible: "I helped my mother to die, at her request, and I am afraid my own death may be earlier than I expected. Though we hardly know each other, I feel that I can ask you to help me to die."

"Archie, what are you asking me to do?" How could he make such a request, I wonder, one so threatening to me, to my professional life? "I don't even know what's wrong with you."

"I am very ill. I have a disease for which there is no known treatment." His head sinks to his chest. He cannot look at me, but I can see tears on his cheeks.

"Felice told me that you looked sick. Your appearance has everyone worried."

"I've tried to maintain normal activity without revealing my condition for the sake of my family. Our finances are very low after my many years in graduate training. I had hoped to be able to work at least for three years in this job." He pauses, unable to go on. He rests his head on his arms on the table. He then sits up and looks anxiously about him, not wanting to make a scene.

He still hasn't named the illness. I wait silently. After a long pause, he explains, "My appointment at the university carries a proviso. I need a physical examination verifying that I am in good health during the first six months of employment in order to assure my family of death benefits." He pauses again. "Without this clearance, I'd have to survive for three years for my family to receive death benefits. But I became ill two months after I arrived here, before any examination was arranged. Now, with my diagnosis and the unexpected, rapid progression of this disease, I won't be able to work or even live the required three years. I don't want to end up paralyzed in an iron lung." He is pale, sweating, and moping his face with difficulty.

I am speechless. Despite his secrecy, I would have expected his university colleagues to offer Archie some help. I feel sorry and angry that no one has come to the aid of this obviously sick man. He continues softly so that diners at adjacent tables cannot overhear our conversation.

"I have not discussed this with anyone, but I can't hide it any longer. Two months after we met, I returned to St. Louis to see my wife Mary and my children. We have moved so often in the course of finishing my degree that Mary and I decided to let our kids finish the school year in St. Louis. I also made an appointment then with my physician because I was alarmed by some peculiar, disturbing physical symptoms. I couldn't clip the nails of my right hand by using clippers in my left hand, for instance, because my left hand was too weak. I couldn't explain this sudden onset of weakness. My doctor promptly referred me to a neurologist who, without any explanation, immediately had me admitted to the hospital," he relates, anxiously glancing around to see if any colleagues are witnessing his distress.

"I was ushered onto the neurology ward, a frightening, chaotic, noisy floor. Patients were screaming, tied to their beds. Some seemed paralyzed, others incoherent and incontinent judging by the smells. Others were bound, picking lint off their blankets and clothing, and secluded in corner chairs. I was horrified and fearful. Would I end up in the same condition? I had no idea what to expect or what the doctors were looking for. After days being kept in ignorance, I was discharged from this horror chamber with the diagnosis of Amyotrophic Lateral Sclerosis, Lou Gehrig's disease. I was told there is no known treatment and that my life expectancy is three to four years."

The dining hall is emptying and none of Archie's colleagues is apparent. As we finish our lunch, I realize with relief that we are almost alone. Archie lowers his head to hide his tears. I place my hand over his at the edge of the table. He speaks again softly, with great sadness. I strain to hear him.

"The rapid progression of my disability convinces me that I will not last the three years. My family will therefore not qualify for insurance benefits. I'm told in the final stages I will not be able to breathe on my own. I will end my life paralyzed, with a respirator, and with brain function cruelly intact because only muscles are affected in this disease, and the brain is not a muscle. I can't ask my wife to help me die. I feel, despite our short relationship, Gert, that I can ask you for help."

I feel affection and profound sympathy for this unfortunate man. I feel my pulse racing and my heart fluttering as often happens when I am stressed. I hope he cannot sense my distress. But I don't know Archie well enough to trust him. Does he understand the implications of his request? My silence seems forever. If I agree to help him and am discovered, I could lose my medical license and end up in jail. I want to say yes, but I cannot respond immediately. I feel great empathy—how could I *not* help him? But how could I take such a chance, endangering my family and myself. I am quiet. Is there any way that I can respond without answering his request?

"Have you seen a physician here at the university?" I ask simply to buy time.

"Yes, and I get the same hopeless response: There is no treatment for this disease."

"What about physiotherapy?" I ask. "Would you be willing to undergo treatment that might help to strengthen your remaining muscles and limbs?" I am surprised at the unusually rapid progression of his disability. I believe that he could be helped by strengthening whatever muscle function remains to relieve the edema and the potential site for infection of his swollen arms and hands.

We part with the understanding that he will contact the local neurologist at the university's medical center, and then we will meet again. I know he will ask again for my help with his plan for suicide, and I have no idea of how I will respond then.

Archie's urgent need for care prompts his family to relocate from St. Louis to Philadelphia quickly. Meeting Mary, Laurie, and Jimmy is a bittersweet experience for me. I am so happy they are here to support Archie, but their distress at his appearance of such rapid deterioration is insurmountable. It's especially difficult for fifteen-year-old Jimmy to adjust to a strange new environment and the impending death of his father. His anguish is reflected in his social withdrawal and slipping schoolwork, but his physical strength is greatly needed by Archie. In the months to come, Archie's physical deterioration becomes primarily Jimmy's burden.

Mary is a strong, sympathetic woman who keeps the family bonded. Laurie immediately hooks up with a boyfriend. Two weeks after Archie's family arrives we met again. He is even more despondent.

"Mary and I went to my internist and got the referral to the physiotherapy department. I paid my fee but when we arrived for the appointment, they not only hadn't received my records but also told us they had nothing to offer me."

So we are forced to devise our own program of activity. Making potholders on a small loom that I provide reduces the swelling of Archie's hands. I am now supplied with enough potholders for years to come. With Jimmy's help, Archie can mount a stationary bike. His leg muscles, which haven't been irretrievably lost, are strengthened by exercise. This improves his gait and reduces the number of falls.

Archie and his family are appreciative and amazed at his progress. They all help to carry out his program and are heartened by the early results. The disease, however, continues to progress very quickly. With the volunteer help of my hospital's Physiotherapy Department, we devise a movable arm brace that functions on ball bearings and allows him to feed himself and even smoke a cigarette. My goal is to keep him as functional as possible, but his rate of deterioration is rapid. When he can no longer make it to the university, Archie's students come to his home for classes.

I am afraid his death is imminent. He certainly cannot last much longer. Then a surprising new hope appears on the horizon— actually on the other side of the globe. Unbeknownst to me at this time, three American doctors visit the People's Republic of China in 1970 as the first Americans to be invited after the visit of President Nixon. Dr. Paul Dudley White, who was President Eisenhower's cardiologist, Dr. E. Gray Dimond of St. Louis Medical School, and Dr. Samuel Rubin, a progressive ear, nose and throat specialist from New York City, are received by the Chinese Medical Association and apprised of the state of medicine in the People's

Republic. They receive a comprehensive review of traditional as well as herbal medicines used in China.

On their return, the three doctors publish an exciting, extensive article in the *Journal of the American Medical Association* (*JAMA*). They describe a presentation by Dr. Hsui Jung about the successful treatment of chronic poliomyelitis with a medication derived from an indigenous plant *securinega suffruticosa* and its derivative *securinine*. Polio destroys the anterior horn cell of the spinal cord, as does ALS. *Chronic* poliomyelitis was not known in the United States in the 1970s. (The type of polio that was eradicated by the Salk vaccine in 1955 was stationary, a one-time paralysis. But chronic poliomyelitis is resurgent; that is, it returns.)

When I read their report in JAMA, I feel cautiously optimistic: Could the Chinese be treating ALS and calling it chronic polio? For the first time since Archie made his anguished disclosure to me, I wonder if we could hope for more than just making the onset his death more comfortable.

18

Archie # 2: Securinega Suffruticosa

Archie is deteriorating rapidly. Statistically he has thirty months left. Are the Chinese in fact treating ALS? Could their herbal medicine be obtained? In my wildest dreams, I hope that Archie might be helped if my premise is correct. When I show the JAMA article to Reuben, my husband, he responds with unaccustomed enthusiasm. "This may be the most important thing you will ever have done in your lifetime," he says.

Reuben's reaction prompts me to show the article to Archie and Mary. I introduce it by warning, "This may be a wild goose chase, but we have nothing to lose." I enlist Mary's most willing help in tracking down the authors. I send a letter of inquiry, introducing myself and outlining the project, to Dr. Dimond in St. Louis. I follow up with a phone call, and thus begins my career, or obsession as it becomes. This compelling project will take up every free moment for years to come. Those years will be absorbing and dramatic.

When I dial St. Louis, his secretary responds, "Dr. Dimond is extremely busy, and he suggests that you contact Dr. Hsui Jung in Beijing."

I cannot reach Dr Jung. Dr. Paul Dudley White and Dr. Rubin, the other authors, are out of town. This is only the first of many unyielding, time-consuming, disappointing dead ends. Library and journal searches for other areas of the world where this plant grows are equally unsuccessful—a daunting, fruitless attempt with my limited resources.

But after the first surge of hope, I cannot face Archie with such bad news. I then remember a good friend since adolescence. Dr. Green, or Dutch to his friends, is a research director at Smith, Kline, and French, a prestigious local pharmaceutical company. In such a position, Dutch has the facilities for an international literature search. (Our local medical libraries have no such accessibility and Internet computer searches are unknown in the early 1970s.)

When I described our project, Dutch gladly offers his services. Archie and Mary are kept informed of our search, but they do not meet Dr. Green until later and under surprising circumstances. Dutch is quickly able to locate the areas of the world where this plant is found: Japan, China, and the northern steppes of the Soviet Union.

When he calls one day, Dutch's voice projects an excitement that only a good researcher can have, "I found a paper on securinine! This is the only article published in the United States medical literature. A naval research group studied securinine for its potential strychnine-like effect. Wouldn't you know they'd be interested in its potential use in chemical warfare? There is no other mention of securinine in any available medical publication."

Dutch is now seduced by our project. He joins in the search and later proves to be a key person in Archie's treatment. William Hinton becomes another important contributor and pivotal person. A handsome, imposing six-foot-eight, with an athletic build and unruly hair, Bill is a world traveler and skier. He is very attracted by my offbeat project when I met him under unusual circumstances.

Bill is a knowledgeable "Sinophile" and former employee of UNRA, a government agency involved in agricultural development in foreign countries. After WWII, Bill was sent as an agronomist to Longbow commune in northern China to advise them about increasing their agricultural output. He was one of the few Americans in China before and during its revolutionary upheaval in 1948. When he returned to the United States in 1952, the State Department impounded his notes on the premise that they contained important secret and subversive material from a communist country. A mutual friend, Joe, organized a group of us to raise funds to sue the State Department for the release of Bill's notes. The suit was successful and the impounded material that was released resulted in the publication of Bill's best seller, *Fanshen: A Documentary of Revolution in a Chinese Village.* After this episode Bill and his family became my patients and friends.

I call on Bill with the hope that, with his contacts, he may be able to help me reach the Chinese Medical Organization. When I tell him of my project and the need to contact the Chinese physicians, he immediately responds, "I have a buddy in Peking, Julian Schuman, a UPI correspondent. I'm sure he is still there, and I'm sure he can help. Call him. Tell him I told you to call."

A great idea—but since I speak no Chinese, Bill's suggestion seems disappointingly unrealistic. How can I place a call to a country with which we have no easy diplomatic relations? I feel this will certainly be a dead end, but I make the call. Looking out my office window at the busy City Line Avenue traffic, I start to dial and think, "This is unreal. What makes me think I can get through by just dialing an overseas operator?

An English-speaking operator answers immediately. "Why are you making this call?" he asks. I am so intimidated that I almost hang up. The operator must sense my fear. He adds, "So many crank calls are being made that we have to screen all calls."

At this my worst fears are confirmed. I think back to an experience twenty years ago. I was visited in the 1950s by the FBI, which was investigating me for subversive activities because I'd voted for the Progressive Party and Henry Wallace. This was the post McCarthy cold war period.

Now, in the 1970s, I suddenly fear that paranoia again. Anyone in contact with a so-called socialist country could be suspect. Why was I pursuing what could very well be a no yield search? How could I chance another visit from 'Pork Pie' capped twin FBI agents? (They always appear in twos.) Would they again ring my doorbell, investigate me as a subversive, and terrify me with their verbal threats as my two young daughters cling to my legs? Would they accuse me of being un-American because I refuse them admission to my house? Why am I endangering my family, my career?

During the outrageous reign of Joe McCarthy, so many people were fired or threatened with jail sentences. Careers were wrecked, families disrupted. Ten of my good friends and patients—several of whom had received awards as outstanding teachers of the year— were fired for incompetence after they appeared in front of the Velde Committee and refused to testify and incriminate their colleagues. Esther and Bill, my neighbors, patients, and emergency baby-sitters, were forced to leave home for several days after the hearings because their house was stoned. Esther had received the award for the best elementary school teacher in the city that year, yet was one of those fired for incompetency! The national atmosphere was frightening and oppressive.

By pursuing this search for an elusive Chinese herbal medicine, am I placing myself in an unpopular, even risky position now, twenty years later? My renewed anxiety is confirmed during one of my calls to Bill at his experimental farm in Bucks County. As one of the first Americans to export wheat to the Soviet Union after the national boycott was lifted, Bill is still on the FBI's surveillance list. I glance out my den window in mid-phone call and spot someone suspended on the telephone pole in my back lawn. He is wearing workman's dark overalls and earphones.

This twilight scene almost derails the project. My face is well lit by my desk lamp, his by the orange glow of the setting sun. For a moment we seem to glare directly at each other. My phone is obviously being tapped. But Archie is deteriorating so rapidly that this scare can have no effect.

Miraculously I reach a Beijing operator who speaks English. I am told that Julian Schuman is not at this particular hotel. There are so few foreigners in Beijing, though, that the operator knows of him, tells me the name of the hotel where he is staying, and puts my call through. At the mention of Bill's name, Julian is willing to help.

"I am not familiar with Dr. Jung," he says, "but I suggest that you try to reach Dr. Hatum, who was Chairman's Mao personal physician on The Long March. He speaks English and is a highly renowned physician of the People's Republic of China. He's a great guy. I'm sure he'll help you."

This sounds like another seemingly impossible route, but I have been lucky so far. I plunge ahead into the unknown. Calls to Beijing reveal that Dr. Hatum is in Switzerland ministering to the famous author and friend of China, Edgar Snow. (Snow is terminally ill and dies shortly after this.) My efforts to reach Dr. Hatum in Switzerland are to no avail. I later learn that he is consoling the widow, Lois Snow, at a secret site somewhere in Zermatt.

I am about to despair when my friend Dutch calls. He sounds elated.

"I found the institute in Moscow where several Russian scientists are working on securinine. Call them, Gert, and see if you can get through."

Calling so-called enemy countries has made me much braver now. I dial the institute directly and reach an English-speaking person who relates that Dr. Knezeva no longer works there. His present location is unknown. Suspicious and distrustful of foreigners, I think. Again I fear that, by calling the Soviet Union, I will be reactivating a political investigation and creating a threat to my family.

I do manage, however, to request information about securinine. And as promised, the Russians send several reprints describing the use of the drug. The mailing somehow reaches my office, addressed only to me in "Philadelphia U.S.A." No street address. The envelope has not been opened. My paranoia takes hold. How did I get this material from the Soviet Union without a street address? Mail, even properly addressed, is often lost in the system. Sleepless nights and anxiety filled days follow, but Archie's deterioration is of greater importance.

These reprints would hopefully hold the promise of dosage and indication for drug use, but the articles are written in Russian. And at this time, the Library of Congress has not a single medical reprint from any of the Eastern European countries, and therefore no translators. So little is known of what is happening in medicine in that large part of our world. A Russian translator is not only prohibitively expensive, but cannot handle scientific material. I am stymied and distraught. Time is running out as Archie wastes away.

I go to see him on a sunny afternoon. He sits in his bedroom with the curtains drawn. He resembles a skeleton, wan, frightening. Each day he looks more like a concentration camp survivor as his nerves and muscles die.

"Gert, I don't know how much longer I can last, or whether I even want to go on. I am such a burden to everyone, especially to Jimmy. The poor kid has to lift me in and out of the bathtub, sit me on the toilet, dress me, and feed me when Mary goes off to work. The students Mary hired to be with me so she can work are depleting whatever funds we have left." I put my arms around his bony shoulders. I am almost afraid I might crush him. I have nothing to say. I simply hold him and sob silently with him.

We are on a magical trail, however. A few days later Mary calls to tell me she met a librarian at the National Library who found a resident Korean librarian who is able to translate the Russian papers. I can scarcely contain my excitement. From this translator, I learn that the Russians had prescribed securinine in a low dose, one-tenth of that used in China, as a potent sexual stimulant for males. In fact, it is available in pill form in pharmacies in the Soviet Union.

I suddenly recall that two of my patients are scheduled to travel to the Soviet Union soon. I call and beg them to bring back some of the pills.

"What will happen to us if we are caught carrying drugs out of a foreign country, especially Russia?" They are alarmed and I can't blame them, but when I tell them about Archie and his terrible disease, and the drug that might conceivably help him to live a little longer, they agree. I suggest that they transfer the pills into one of their own empty pill bottles. They do so and encounter no difficulty.

They return with the pills but no information about dosage. The only information accompanying the pills concerns their use for sexual impotence. This, in fact, is one of Archie's symptoms, and it will later prove to be significant. The dosage and purity of the pills become our immediate concerns: How to determine the purity of the pills? How much it is safe to use? How much might produce convulsions? It is essential to get the drug in purer form than pills.

Phil, a long time friend, calls from New York to chat. When I describe my project, he reminds me that our mutual friend, Gibby, travels frequently to Russia. Gibby is an attorney who has been employed for many years by NewYork-based Amtorg, a Russian agency that controls imports and exports for Russia. Gibby might be able to help me.

When I reach Gibby, he is his usual direct self, "Do you mean Russia has something in medicine that we don't have? I don't believe it!" I talk excitedly about my project, and he agrees to bring back whatever information and/or drug he can find. He knows I am somewhat of a maverick.

Another wonderful unexpected development: Archie's wife Mary has a friend in Washington who works with the International Research and Exchange Board (IREX). This friend puts us in contact with Dan Matuszewski, a Princeton University professor, who directs the IREX project. Dan is in charge of the exchange of postdoctoral biophysics graduate students from the Soviet Union and has many international contacts.

Mary and I visit him at his home in Princeton to explain our quest. He quickly understands the urgency of our cause and responds immediately. As we watch and listen, Dan picks up the phone and calls his agent in Moscow. He instructs him to hunt down the drug and bring some back in his diplomatic pouch.

Transport in the diplomatic pouch will insure its delivery without examination and possible delay.

Two weeks later Mary meets the courier in Washington. He delivers three dozen vials of securinine in solution—the pure material in sterile solution we want! But unfortunately, the package contains no information describing its concentration and /or frequency of administration. Nevertheless this cache is a real windfall and will prove to be very important in Archie's initial treatment.

During this same time period, Professor Matuszewski contacts his representative in Japan who is able to bring back seeds of the plant within a month. As soon as I receive the seeds, I approach Dr. John Fogg, an agronomist and director of the Horticultural School at the Barnes Foundation in Merion. He is instantly excited by my story and responds almost gleefully, "You know, Doctor, my primary interest and research has been in the field of herbal medicine. I was in the group that brought the first plant treatment of hypertension to our country."

(Dr. Fogg was indeed one of two investigators who successfully developed the first drug treatment for high blood pressure—hypertension—used in the United States. It was derived from the plant *Rauwolfia Serpentina*, *Reserpine*, discovered during WWII in India where it was grown and used to treat high blood pressure. Dr. Fogg then cultivated the plant in Puerto Rico, but the procedure to derive the drug from the farm product proved too expensive. Dr. Fogg and his associate were able to synthesize the drug in the laboratory, which was cheaper than growing it in the field.)

Dr. Fogg needs little persuasion. "Come, I have something to show you in the arboretum," he says, leading me to the site where he grows *securinega* that he imported from China years ago as an exotic plant. Its medicinal potential was unknown to him. I am amazed that this precious plant, which I've been tracking down on the other side of the world, is actually growing in an arboretum within walking distance of my home.

Dr. Fogg enthusiastically joins our project and becomes a valuable ally. I feel very lucky and encouraged by his response. In the Barnes Foundation greenhouse, he cultivates the seeds we've just received from Japan. I then transplant the seedlings in my back lawn and on my brother Eddie's farm in Burlington, New Jersey, where they continue to thrive.

Dr. Fogg also informs me that, before retiring from University of Pennsylvania where he was the acting director of the Morris Arboretum, he had planted a *securinega* plant in its exotica section. With this news, I set off to find it. While my friends shield me, I crawl under the bush and whack off several branches. But I am later unsuccessful in propagating them. (In spite of my vandalism, the bush is still flourishing when I revisit it thirty years later.)

Although we are making progress in procuring *securinega*, we still have not been able to translate the Russian material that potentially holds the key to treatment—until once again, help comes from an unexpected source. I'm invited to a friend's house, where I meet two Russian postdoctoral biophysicists assigned to work in Burton Chance's bio-research laboratory at the University of Pennsylvania. As usual, the conversation centers around my project. Either my friends are supportive and encouraging, or I am just irrepressible! The Russian students speak English fluently and are enthusiastic and curious.

"We would be delighted to help you translate the papers. The project sounds exciting!" They invite me to bring the Russian articles to their laboratory some Sunday evening. Buoyed by this fortuitous offer, I arrive at the deserted campus on a wintry Sunday evening. The only visible lights are in their laboratory at the far corner of the building—a perfect cloak and dagger scene. Here I am, at night in a deserted building, meeting two scientists from a communist country. Apprehensively I enter the huge darkened building and expect to be accosted at any moment by an armed guard or some other assailant in the empty corridor. I am ready to call out for help as I hurry through the unlit hall. With a sigh of relief, I burst into their laboratory.

"What's wrong? You look so upset," they greet me.

"The building is so empty and dark." I am determined to ask them to walk me out when I leave.

These two tall foreigners and I perch on high stools where my feet dangle, barely reaching the first rung. I feel like a midget between them in size and intellect. They translate the material and describe in detail the parenteral use of the drug, i.e., the material in solution by injection. They translate the Russian directions, and I the medical alliterative terms.

Now we have the medication in vials and in injectable form brought in by the IREX messenger, as well as the recommended dosage translated by the two Russian students. But we do not know the concentration of the drug in the Soviet ampoules or how to determine this. We are fearful that, in our ignorance, we might cause a convulsion. We need more information from China about the precise dosage, if it is being used in the People's Republic of China, and for what purpose. Direct contact with the Chinese Medical Association has to be established. But how? Once again I feel out of my depth.

Though the People's Republic of China does not yet have an embassy in the United States, it does have an official delegation housed in a New York City hotel. Bill Hinton informs the delegation of our project and the pressing need to contact the Chinese Medical Association. He travels with me to New York, introduces me to the officials, and accompanies me on many subsequent trips. The delegation accepts and trusts me because I am introduced by their respected friend. I am overwhelmed.

We met in a large hotel room that appears to be a bedroom without a bed. I enter with Bill to meet a silent, serious group of twelve men and women in western dress. Most speak only Chinese. I feel alien until Bill translates their warm greeting. They, as the only representatives of this government of close to 900 million people, accept me in their headquarters! Bill is certainly their trusted and honored friend, and Archie is in this way a lucky patient.

The delegation contacts the Chinese Medical Association directly and explains Archie's situation and our search. From this point on, whenever we communicate, members of the delegation and representatives of the medical association in China solicitously inquire about the professor and his illness. In all the numerous phone calls for information or translation of material, whoever answers the phone—from secretaries to highly placed delegates—everyone always asks about Archie's condition. I feel that our two countries are involved in a non-political humanitarian project.

Each visit to New York is like entering another world. Some delegates speak English. Bill translates for others. I feel honored to be admitted to this inner sanctum, and I am continually amazed at our good fortune in this unbelievable, uncharted territory. These events also occur before the introduction and general acceptance of alternative and herbal medicine. We do not yet have a department at the National Institutes of Health to evaluate or even recognize alternative and herbal medicine. I therefore am reluctant to discuss our project with my most of my medical colleagues.

In spite of our unprecedented successes, we are constantly aware of Archie's rapid deterioration. His time is running out, and we are still stymied, not sure of the dose, and fearful of making him worse in our ignorance.

Dutch Green then discovers a gold mine: His company has some securinine saved in its vault for possible future research needs. We still aren't sure of the purity, potency, or concentration of the material in the ampoules, our only 'pure' source, nor do we know how to test for its properties because the chemistry is still unknown to us. Dutch appeals to his company to release some of its drug, two grams of which it has in solid form. We could titrate it to determine its potency. The head of research agrees to release one-half gram, either for humanitarian reasons or because Dutch is held in such esteem. Whatever the reason, we feel lucky to have the medication available so quickly, as we are to discover shortly.

From the Russian literature translated by the two postgraduate students, we have determined some dosage and frequency of administration. From Dutch we have a quantifiable amount, and from the Chinese we have the dose they are using in what they call chronic polio. We now know approximately how much to use.

Now that we have the promise of the drug and the plants from which it could be extracted, my husband Reuben and Dr. Ara Der Marderosian, who both work at the School of Pharmacology, become vitally involved. Reuben is responsible for the actual drug treatment of Archie, Dr. Marderosian for the derivation of the drug from its plant. Ready for the first trial, we are anxious and fearful, but Archie and his family have no hesitation. They are eager to try anything as soon as possible.

Archie has been having some difficulty breathing and swallowing but does not reveal this to his wife or to me. He knows that these bulbar symptoms signify end-stage disease, and he is fearful that this new development could interfere with our experimental administration of the drug. He is determined to receive the drug and chance any adverse effects because he hopes not to end his life on a respirator. Archie has also developed footdrop, which makes walking difficult. He walks very slowly now and climbs stairs by placing both feet on each step.

We hospitalize Archie for the initial administration of the drug because we fear the possible strychnine-like response of inducing convulsions. We want Archie under close supervision. (At this time, in the early 1970s, we are allowed to use an experimental drug under such circumstances with just a government license. This is notably before the proliferation of malpractice legal terror.)

His family gather in his hospital room. Mary, Jimmy, and Laurie each embrace Archie and exchange whispered messages. Then they stand silently, holding hands. Around his bed in this small hospital room, we've amassed a pile of emergency equipment: IV poles, respirator, shock pads, all sorts of life-saving material, should a convulsion or any other adverse reaction take place. We surround the bed as he receives his first dose. A neurologist, Dr. Myron Fredericks, medical students, floor nurses, and three investigators stand by, anxious and ready to pounce if necessary but not really knowing what to expect. Archie is the calmest in the crowd.

The first doses, given by mouth, are of a smaller dosage and more readily controlled. After the first few oral doses given over three days with no adverse effects, we give him the first injection, a small amount, with no visible change. On the sixth day after the third injection, Archie smiles and says in a stronger than usual voice, "I did not tell anyone that I had some difficulty swallowing and breathing for the last few days before hospital admission. Now these symptoms have disappeared almost completely after the first three injections."

His family and the attendants surrounding his bed hug each other. We couldn't all hug Archie! These results are beyond our wildest dreams. Archie's footdrop also disappears. We walk him out to the stairway of the indoor fire escape and he can manage stairs without placing both feet on each step before advancing up or down. He can now walk one stair at a time. The footdrop and bulbar symptoms, the breathing and swallowing problems all disappear, never to return in his life span. For Archie, his family, and the attendant medical personnel, there is exultation in his remarkable, almost unbelievable response!

19

Archie # 3: Securinega Suffruticosa

Archie's goal has been to live and teach for three years so that his family can receive death benefits. With the amazing results in his early treatment, Archie and his family's expectations soar. In the spring before he received the medication, he had been distressed by the resurgence of life in nature while he simultaneously and rapidly advanced towards death. Now he is able to enjoy the drive through Fairmount Park and revel in the flowering magnolias and dogwood. The disappearance of the breathing and swallowing problems—the bulbar symptoms that mark the end stage of the disease—was wonderfully hopeful.

And there is an unexpected added benefit. During one of Archie and Mary's visits, we're sitting in our back yard and Archie is beaming. In his usual direct way, he tells my husband Reuben and me, "Mary and I have had sex several times since I returned home from the hospital."

He pauses at our vociferous response.

"You know, previously, despite Mary's efforts, I wasn't able to have an erection for many months prior to the treatment. I remember your telling me, from the Russian literature, that the drug was a sexual stimulant. We certainly proved it." There were broad grins on all our faces. Mary and Archie are able to enjoy intercourse for many more months.

Archie's new pleasures, the lifting of his depression and resentment, and his good humor reverberate through his family and circle of friends. His strength increases. Color replaces his deathly pallor. After the first few weeks of the drug, he announces, "Gert, I'm ready to go back to the classroom." In my wildest dreams, I never expected to hear this.

After his initial remarkable response, however, Archie's condition does not continue to improve, but neither does it deteriorate. We adjust our expectations and are pleased that he holds steady for several months. During this time Archie's experience with the medical profession in general is abominable. He is treated unsympathetically and often made to feel stupid and inadequate. He has not only been teaching during the course of his disease but has also published a book, *Notes of a Dying Professor*, in addition to several articles on the disease and his treatment.

On one of my many house calls and drop-ins, I find Archie unusually angry.

"Gert, you would not believe what I was subjected to this past week! A medical colleague asked me to appear in front of his class to demonstrate my rare disease to his students. He insisted that I be wheeled in even though I obviously can still walk."

Archie's eyes are bright with unshed tears. "My protests had no effect. I almost refused, but I thought my presentation would be valuable for the students. This was unbearably insulting to me." He stops and tries to control his wavering voice. Wringing his hands, he continues, "They treated me as if I was an inanimate object. They looked at me, discussed my condition, then promptly wheeled me out. There was a lot I could have told them about the inconsiderate and inhumane treatment that a dying person receives at the hands of the helping profession."

His anger is palpable. I am horrified at the insensitivity of my colleagues. This is so uncomfortable for Archie, who is usually so grateful and uncomplaining.

"On several hospital admissions, because my movements are so slow, I am awakened at six in the morning instead of at seven, when the other patients are awakened. They receive their breakfast at 8 A.M. and, though I am up earlier, I'm not served until 9 A.M. I finally complained and the time was changed, which evoked a snide remark from the floor nurse. She actually asked me if I enjoyed the extra hour of sleep. I felt incompetent and stupid."

During this period Archie's disease advances but at a slower rate than before. His breathing and swallowing remain intact. His daily life assumes almost a satisfactory pattern. He teaches his classes at the university and enjoys his family and the splendid Philadelphia springtime.

Then late one afternoon, I receive an emergency call from Mary. "This last injection didn't work. Archie can't even sit up."

We assume that something must be wrong with this new batch of medicine. I dash over with a fresh batch of securinine. Archie is lying prostrate on a cot. I give him a shot of the fresh material and in less than twenty minutes, he miraculously stands up and walks the length of his house. With Archie recovered, I prepare to leave. Mary walks me to the door. She looks so sad. I try to reassure her.

"There must have been something wrong in the preparation, Mary. I'm sure he will be okay." I put my arms around her as she sobs quietly. "I'm sure that was just a bad batch. Toss out the rest of it, and I'll bring over more fresh preparation tomorrow."

I leave them to attend a party at a friend's house. I arrive to find the house full—it's a surprise fiftieth birthday party for me. Sitting in the circle of friends, the greatest surprise of all is a beaming Archie with Mary beside him.

"Oh, my gosh, how did you make it?"

"That last shot was miraculous" Archie grins, "But I would have come in a wheelchair if I had to."

Archie does relatively well for about a year and a half on the drug. Some deterioration occurs, but compared to his rapid disability at the disease's onset, this is slower than it would have been without the medication. The last several months of the semester, as he becomes weaker, his students again come to his house for class. Near the end of this last school term when he is much weaker, his voice becomes soft and quavering. Mary reports, "I have been giving him an injection just before the class so his voice can be heard for the hour of lecture." Mary begins to sob, "He's failing."

With the administration of securinine, Archie survives the three years required for health and insurance benefits. Judging from his prior history with the disease, we believe that without securinine his life would have ended earlier. Archie requires total care toward the end. He refuses all treatment except for essential support and comfort. He dies at 3 A.M. one month after the semester ends. I help him to die with dignity.

When I leave Archie and return home, my husband reports that at 3 A.M., he suddenly awoke from a sound sleep and sat bolt upright in bed. I lie awake for the rest of this night and many more. Archie's struggle has ended, but I review the three years since we first met. I'm haunted by the deterioration of this brilliant, brave, vibrant man who became a paralyzed skeleton but whose mind remained cruelly alert—his brain imprisoned, the last functioning part of himself. And what bravery his family showed over those last three years.

Our work with Archie and securinine was reported and published in a medical journal, but it excited little response. No pharmaceutical company could make any profit with this medication because so few people are alive with this disease.

Thirty years after Archie's death, my daughter calls to tell me of an obscure government statement that somehow I have missed. An unusually heavy incidence of ALS has been reported among veterans of the first Gulf War of 1991.

I remember Archie's plant and feel that I need to save it for some potentially important use. I have not seen the plant in many years, and I fear that I would not recognize it. Yet I return to the Morris Arboretum with my friend Alice, a horticulturist. We search but cannot find the securinine plant. I am sure we are at the proper site, but nothing looks familiar. Have they moved the plant? Has it died? Has it changed so after thirty years that I can't recognize it? My knowledgeable friend Alice suggests, "Let's go to the library. It must have a map of all these plantings."

The library is not open to the public this day, but the librarian graciously leads us into his office and clicks on his computer when we explain our quest. We discover that we do not recognize the plant because it has grown into a small tree. We also learn that securinine is now described as a medicinal plant in horticultural literature. It is used in China and Japan to treat multiple sclerosis and certain spinal cord injuries when the cord has been contused but not severed. With administration of the drug, they have demonstrated movement in atrophied muscles at the level of the injury. Securinine is listed as one of the thirty most used medications in China and Japan.

With the government reports today of an unusual number of ALS patients connected to the first Gulf War, securinine might offer some help. And Archie's story might be an impetus for further research and a ray of hope for ALS patients and those suffering from spinal cord contusions.

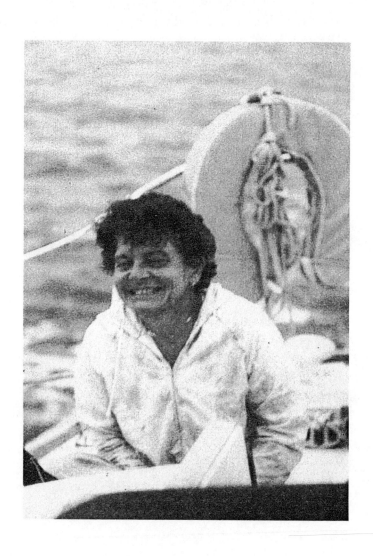

20

Hostile Currents

Threatening overcast skies, mackerel clouds, gusting winds, swirling leaves -the end of summer with its variable weather. But we are not discouraged. After five days of pelting rains, playing checkers and chess, reading and overeating, we have to get outside on this first rain-free day.

I have to swim. This is my last day on the island of Martha's Vineyard. I'm flying out tomorrow. Making light of the possible storm, we set sail from our lake out to the sound. I can't swim in our Lake Tashmoo because invading Canada geese have taken it over. Huge green swaths of feces cover the lake's surface. Diving in would result in more than a mouthful of water.

The wind grows stronger, clouds darker, water rougher. Sails are luffing as we pass through the narrow inlet to the clean waters of the sound. Our plans change. Under the present conditions, it's foolhardy to travel to a more distant area to swim in a protected cove. Skipper Saul drops anchor instead, just a little further out into open clear water of the sound.

We are anxious to swim before the rain, but we neglect to check the current, an unusual oversight by Saul, the ultimate compulsive skipper. I jump in as soon as Jenny throws overboard the floating buoy that is tied to the boat. The current swiftly carries me away like a piece of flotsam. I cannot swim back to the boat. With great difficulty, I can just about swim in place. I struggle with all my strength to keep the current from carrying me still further out into deeper waters. I start to wheeze. I become frantic. I have exercised harder than this in the past without wheezing. I become breathless—am I going into heart failure? I have no chest pain, but it is becoming harder to breathe. I flail frantically, beating the water. I can't allow myself to panic. If I do, I will surely drown. I trust Saul. I know he will rescue me, but how?

"Stay afloat," he yells to me, as if I have a choice. But Saul is encouraging: "I'm coming." He barely has to swim. The current swiftly carries him toward me.

"Grab hold of my foot. I'll pull you in."

The current is stronger than Saul, and we make no progress "Let go, but keep pumping. I'll swim to that beach to get help," he says reassuringly.

I reluctantly let go of his foot. Then the swift current miraculously delivers the cushion that Jenny has thrown in. It reaches and rescues me. What a relief! With all my remaining strength, I climb onto the cushion. I'm then lying on the surface of the water, and the current has less effect. I slowly kick my way into the shallow water. I can see Saul on the nearby beach where he's running frantically, looking for help. There's an overturned rowboat, without oars, and not a person or house on the deserted beach.

I kick my way toward Saul, who is now standing and waiting in water that's fenced in by huge rocks that jut out like two piers. When I reach him, we're neck deep in the calm water of this protected pocket. We feel safer than we did twenty minutes ago, but we're nevertheless stranded on an unpopulated beach and a storm is coming.

We can get onto the beach if necessary, but Jenny is unable to manage the boat alone. Even more worrisome, she is an insulin-dependent diabetic whose medications occasionally do not control her disease. I cannot see Jenny on deck. Is she already in trouble? I feel guilt ridden. Were it not for me, the boat would have stayed anchored at Lake Tashmoo in this weather.

Saul and I are protected from the current in this protected spot, but we're unable to swim out to where the boat is anchored.

"What in the world do we do now, Saul?" My teeth are chattering, I'm getting colder, but we can't move out. Saul puts his arms around me for reassurance and warmth.

"Jenny will get help," he says, trying to reassure me. (I do not realize that Jenny has called the Coast Guard. She knows what to do in an emergency. She and Saul have experienced several in their travels. Once they missed their port in Connecticut because of fog and were lost somewhere off the Rhode Island coast. Jenny was running out of insulin and a call to the Coast Guard produced her rescue.)

The Coast Guard's response is amazingly quick. Three boats appear to rescue us. A fourth boat, that of the harbor master of Lake Tashmoo, has picked up the distress signal from Jenny and is now tying up to her boat, to stand by should she need help.

On the largest boat, we can see eight men ringing the deck and peering at us through glasses. They are apparently ready to jump in if we appear to be in trouble. We are not in danger if we stay here. But we cannot get out into deeper water because of the current, and the boats are too large to come in over the submerged rocks and between the rocky piers.

A fifth vessel soon appears. We are still standing and shivering in neck-deep water while five boats float out there. The fifth fortunately is a raft with no keel, so it can motor in close enough to throw out life buoys that can reach us despite the opposing current. Our rescuers drag us on the buoys through the water to the larger boat—we are water-skiing without the skis! After we're hauled aboard, we are examined, but we've suffered no injuries. The Coast Guard takes our names and addresses and carries us back to Jenny.

As we climb on board, Jenny says, "Look up."

A helicopter circles above, flown out all the way from Woods Hole to aid in our rescue. Five boats and a helicopter—never have I felt so important. Our rescue is reported on the radio and in the local papers. Amazing how many people, so many miles away, read *The Vineyard Gazette*.

My daughters are appalled but not surprised.

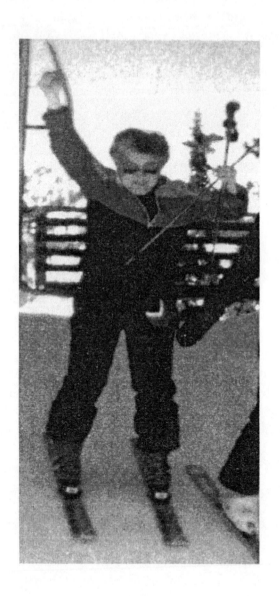

21

Hot Chili on a Cold Day

My policy is always to eat a very light lunch when skiing, but the chili smells *so* good. The day is bitingly cold and menacingly windy, as often happens here at Snowbird in this Utah canyon. The chili is warming and delicious. I eat a huge bowlful. It's late in the day, the winter sun will soon be setting, and my buddy, who is impatient to get in the last runs, insists, "Come on, Gert. Let's go!"

"Wait a sec. Let me at least swallow the last mouthful."

Barely waiting for me to put on my skis, he starts off. I catch up to him on the next chair—for a trip that is to end in disaster.

We start down together. But the trail winds around, and I manage to lose him by taking a wrong turn on the very first run. I shout for him. No response. I'm on top of a steep hill with no sign of a trail through the trees. Everything is wiped out by the swirling snow. How am I going to get down? I am alone in deep powder, a forest of trees, and no ski lift to follow down.

The sun is fast setting under heavy layers of clouds. The wind swirls the surface snow. Hard icy pellets hit my cheeks. I hate facemasks, but I sure wish I had one now. I try never to ski alone, but I have no choice now and I'm scared. The powder is too deep to try to hike down. I have no idea where I am, but I know I have to get down or freeze. I am certain that the ski patrol will not be sweeping this ungroomed, unskied area.

I fall several times, lose a ski, and have to dig down into the snow for it. My fingers feel frost bitten because I have to remove my outer mittens to reattach the skis. Icy water drips from my nose. My eyes are smarting and my glasses are frosting up. I ski, slide, scramble, and roll most of the way down the hill.

Finally reaching the bottom, I don't know where I've landed. But I'm thankful to see a plowed, paved flat road ahead. I don't know if I am heading away from or towards the lodge. I walk about one-half mile and find a parking lot, but it's not the one attached to my lodge. This one, as I soon discover, is two miles from mine. I have traveled some distance!

The sun is now setting and the temperature is easily ten degrees lower than when I started the day. People are packing up and loading into their cars. Everyone is rushing, hungry, exhausted, and wet from snow and sweat. Cars are full of people and equipment. I don't recognize anyone, but I must look as badly as I feel, shivering, wet, and weary. Some people take pity on me when I tell them I'm lost. They load me and my gear into an already packed car. They drive two miles out of their way back to my lodge. Skiers are the friendliest gang of folks.

When we arrive at my lodge, they want to carry my gear up for me. But I have defrosted a bit and can manage alone. I share a room but not a bed, with Jack, my friend's present heartthrob, because she could not make this trip. I am shivering, curled up under a pile of blankets, when he finally arrives.

"What happened to you? Where did you turn off?" Jack asks impatiently.

"I lost you on the hill. Why didn't you stop to look for me instead of just skiing off? You were skiing too fast for me to follow you. Why didn't you wait for me to catch up?" Almost sobbing, I am angry and feeling sorry for myself.

My speech suddenly becomes garbled. Jack continues to talk to me, but I am floating in and out of consciousness. I am aware of his calling his girlfriend Ann, a psychiatrist back in Philadelphia, for advice.

"Call 911 for help," she instructs him.

In the ambulance, I hear some spurts of conversation with the technicians, but I still float in and out on the thirty mile ride down the canyon to the nearest hospital.

After five hours of blood tests, CAT scan, and examination by a neurologist, my mental state suddenly clears completely. The wonderful staff neurologist brings a library textbook to my bedside and reads to me the diagnosis: transient amnesia. "Transient" is small consolation. This is still a frightening diagnosis. How soon will it recur? How do I get home to Philadelphia?

An ambulance transports me the back to the lodge at 4:30 A.M. I arrange to be met with a wheelchair in Denver, where I have to change planes, and in Philadelphia by my daughter.

An explanation: Hot chili draws blood away from the brain to the stomach for digestion; this results in decreased blood supply to an already aged brain.

Ever since this experience, my lunches consist of hot chocolate and packages of peanut butter crackers. All around me, I notice others enjoying steaming bowls of chili, delicious pasta, hot soups, and wine. I make up for this deprivation at dinner.

The likelihood of a recurrent episode is very low, yet for several years I am afraid to travel alone. But as happens after all my other calamitous events, my anxiety is gradually relieved because there's no recurrence. I ski, but rarely alone. I did get lost once last year, again in a sudden snow squall. It was the end of the day, and I made one last run.